BREAST MILK:

Infant Nurture For Best Outcomes

from

THEODORA EKWEVUGBE, MD

To,

DR VIVEK PATIL

19/04/2023

Wednesday 09:10

Book Design by Aeyshaa

DEDICATION

Are you are a mum who's searching for the best way to give her child a good start in life? Then this book is for you.

It's my hope that through the stories written here, you will become wiser and have a more realistic view of the expectations along your breastfeeding journey; that you will see why it is all so worth it, and why if given a choice in retrospect, you wouldn't have had it any other way.

I want you to know that despite whatever challenges you may face, you are doing the right thing by choosing to breastfeed your child.

CONTENTS

ACKNOWLEDGMENT

To my husband, Tobore Ekwevugbe, thanks for giving me the opportunity, support, and environment to write this book. Thank you for believing in me, encouraging me, and giving me the support to go after my dreams. I appreciate it. Thank you.

To my children, Nathan and Esther, who've allowed me the opportunity to pass through the things I did, and by so doing, garner the experience that has produced this book, I say thanks.

To all the mums (Ifeoluwa Dare, Tosin Kehinde, Tosin Idowu, Dolapo Ajayi, and Dr Kelechi Anyanwu), who shared their experiences, and by doing so provided witness testimonies that identify with some problems that have prompted me to write this book, thanks again for taking the time and lending your voice.

And to the skilful editor, who helped turn my manuscript into a book, Efeturi Ifoghale, thank you so much. You created great ease in the journey to make this happen.

INTRODUCTION

Dear mama or mama-to-be, it's lovely to see you have this book in your hand. You know, breastmilk was the only suitable food made for human babies. It is the specie specific milk for our babies – human babies. Once we establish this, the focus of the learning should then be on establishing women with the knowledge and experience/skill they need to breastfeed their babies expertly and successfully.

God gave every species a suitable means to feed its young. God designed human milk to feed human babies and to provide for the specific needs of a human, including the mental/intellectual needs, physical needs, psychological needs and so on, by the breastfeeding process. Those needs are not all covered for the newborn stage in the nutrition provided by other forms of milk; for example in the cow milk. This is so as cow babies do not need all that we humans do. It is also important to note that breastfeeding is not just about giving breastmilk to the baby; rather, it is also for bonding/tying the mother to her baby, and accomplishing something psychologically profound and needed in the heart and mind of both the mother and her developing baby. It is therapeutic for both mother and child.

This book aims to empower you as a mum to know you are in THE place of authority to parent your children. God gave this role and responsibility to YOU. He also furnishes you with all you need if you ask Him and look to him for answers, just like the answers you will see in this book. You, mum, are the right guardian, and you have the place of authority over decision-making for your child – until they are of age, so take this authority back from every other authority trying to take it away from you. The creator built you intuitively for this and you know what to do (even though it may not always feel like it).

I hope that by the end of this book, you would have a well-furnished mindset, built up with a better understanding of both the important nature and purpose of breastfeeding, and why it is your right and conferred responsibility to choose what is right for your babe.

Lots of love.

CHAPTER 1
MY FIRST EXPERIENCE

My First Child:

I was young when I had my first child. I'm going to describe the mindset I had before and at the time of having my first child, and gradually show you how this changed; because for me, my mindset determined the outcome – whether success or failure of my journey.

Here's the mindset I had to work with the first time around:

Limiting thoughts and beliefs about myself

I was very young and my knowledge limited. Stories of those around me had influenced my expectations. The friend who had to labour hours and hours and still ended up having a caesarean section; those who opted for caesarean section from the onset, rather than even go through the possibility of a failed labour; and those who declined to breastfeed or to breastfeed long, i.e., beyond a few months only, because they were afraid of losing the integrity of the structural architecture of their breasts from breastfeeding multiple children or prolonged breastfeeding with one child. For me, I didn't trust my body to produce the milk I needed. I see this is a fear many others also seem to have.

What we believe about our bodies and our expected breast-feeding outcome, has a dominant influence on how things eventually play out. A breastfeeding journey that will be successful starts with a belief in your ability to do it, and a will to do it. You also need a will to persevere against obstacles, because there may be some. This is one thing I feel so many people lack. Personally, I also lacked in this area.

> *What we believe about our bodies and our expected breastfeeding outcome, has a dominant influence on how things eventually play out. A breastfeeding journey that will be successful starts with a belief in your ability to do it, and a will to do it.*

Surrounding Environment

Being surrounded by people who believe that you can do it is influential and can balloon your chances of success. These people may not be in immediate proximity to you, but should be in 'phone callable' or 'textable' distance. On the other hand, being surrounded by people who have a mindset open to giving up at the first roadblock or resistance, and who hold in their beliefs that formula feeding is equal to breast milk, will reduce your chance of succeeding with breastfeeding.

> *Being surrounded by people who believe that you can do it is influential and can balloon your chances of success.*

I had a healthy, uneventful pregnancy the first time, and when time drew near for labour/delivery; that is my late 3rd trimester, I had concerns about labour and delivery; even breastfeeding. Someone had jokingly asked me if I thought the baby could pass through my pelvis. A friend had also narrated her recent labour experience. She had needed to have a C/S after a prolonged labour. I had looked at my breasts, which appeared reasonably small to me, and I had wondered if these could hold enough milk for the coming baby. Though I know you could properly breast-feed your child independent of breast storage capacity. All these thoughts flooded my mind day in day out with doubts whether I could do this.

On one of my maternity visits in the late trimester, I had curiously asked the midwife out of concern, if I could have a caesarean section instead. I had asked this because I was becoming anxious about labour and delivery. Comments from people had planted a seed in my heart, and I had begun to have doubts whether my baby could pass. She unceremoniously said "no." I had wondered if my asking for it was not enough reason to have it. She said I had no indication (i.e., no medical necessity) to have a C/S. I also asked her if I could carry some bottles of formula to the hospital with me. I wanted to because I was concerned about lactation, and she said "yes." So, I did.

I had no real experience-based information on what I could expect with starting to breastfeed. Beyond the limited information I had from medical training, I did not know what challenges I might face along the way, and what to do with them. Of course, I would have been able to recognise and respond to symptoms of mastitis, or other medical conditions, but things like: the sleep deprivation, searching through different breastfeeding positions to find one that doesn't feel like you're going to lose some of your nipple to the baby's mouth, cluster feeding and being able to tell it's because of a growth spurt and not that you're not producing enough milk to fill the baby at once, were all hidden information to me. As a doctor, and a new one at the time of my pregnancy with my first child, I had not been exposed in practise to women having breastfeeding challenges or those starting their breastfeeding journeys. And this was in part because of my chosen specialty of work at the time – an acute medical ward. I didn't think about how easy or difficult it would be. I certainly didn't know to expect the pain I had with breastfeeding; the woeful pain.

Not everyone's journey will be painful, I know, but mine was, and because I wasn't expecting it or aware it could even be that painful in any circumstance, I had no amount of mental preparation to go through it. So, I gave up as I didn't see a way through. This is part of what this book hopes to accomplish; to show you the way I saw through this, and the other woes one might be blindsided by. If my body and breasts had a mind and feelings of their own, I wonder how sad and put down all those thoughts must have made them feel, considering the human hosting them did not have any confidence in their ability to perform in their God-given roles. This breaks my heart now because of what I have since learnt.

This is part of what this book hopes to accomplish; to show you the way I saw through this, and the other woes one might be blindsided by.

Lastly, talking about factors that made it difficult the first time, there was a lack of the support I needed around me. I didn't know what I needed or what would have helped to make the journey successful, but now, looking back, I realise I didn't have the support I would have used around me. I realise I knew I wanted to breastfeed, but didn't know HOW to breastfeed. There is a skill needed for breastfeeding. Some people get this as it just happens naturally, because of instinct, and they learn as they go. But for a person who lacks confidence in their ability to do the very things, this can feel like a right-handed person learning to write left-handed. It felt awkward. I felt shame and some guilt for not knowing how to do it properly. I believed I had tried my best, so I shielded myself from any further exposure to those feelings. I didn't believe there was anyone to empathise and give me non-judgemental advice at this time. It's worrying how defensive we get when we face situations that potentially expose us to guilt and shame, and how this defensive posture can limit us from getting the information and help we need from those around us who are willing to help us. Not everyone is trying to cause you to feel shame. The guilt may be a response from your human nature due to your not performing an act God built you to perform. I think everyone might feel this if they were in such a situation; unless, of course, they've lost sensitivity to their human feelings.

It's worrying how defensive we get when we face situations that potentially expose us to guilt and shame, and how this defensive posture can limit us from getting the information and help we need from those around us who are willing to help us.

I was also not aware of books written on breastfeeding which gave a guide, provided information, and served as a companion to many women who were also in my situation. I realise now they exist, even though a few. This just describes my state of mind at the start of my first journey, and I have taken the time to outline it all with its gloom, so that you see what I had to work with, and what produced the results I had. I also hope to show you the mindset change I went through, going from that to where I have now come, and to see how each change in my thoughts and beliefs about myself led me through a more victorious journey with much more interesting experiences and encounters, as you will see in subsequent chapters.

How my first breastfeeding journey eventually played out

I took some formula with me to the hospital 'just in case'. Very wrong.

Suggestion: This is wrong because when you determine to pursue a cause, from the onset, you don't leave an opportunity open that encourages you to slip onto another course, 'just in case' you fail at pursuing the chosen cause. This shows an unhelpful double-mindedness, and even worse, it limits your ability for mental toughness and doggedness. Therefore, don't do it. If you have chosen to breastfeed, be prepared to turn down apparently harmless suggestions to bottle feed formula; especially if they are without 'just cause'.

I took some formula with me to the hospital 'just in case'. Very wrong.

I ended up using the formula because:

1. At the hospital, he didn't seem to get much milk out from the breast on sucking.

2. I was impatient. I hadn't realised what I was experiencing in the moment was normal and expected, and so I gave him the formula which was with me. I said to myself, "Rather than watch him starve just because I'm struggling with breastfeeding, I'll be doing what's best for him by letting him have some formula." How far I was from the truth. **Now, I realise that's the mindset for 'fed is best.' The issue here wasn't a genuine need for alternative feeding methods, but an ignorance of what was normal and expected at this stage.**

I had bought the pre-made up (Liquid) formula bottles, which were easy to administer, and this was what I ended up using throughout my breastfeeding journey. This cost us a lot of money. I did this as I didn't want to suffer any complications of not properly reconstituting the powder formulation, and also the greater hygiene risks. Because of the above, I didn't put him to the breast as much. When we tried, the latch was difficult to establish, and painful. I successfully nursed him from my nipples on some occasions when my milk came in. And each time, it thrilled me we could do it. But this wasn't often. In my case, it was more painful than I could have imagined. I cried. I don't think I cried during my labour, but I cried during breastfeeding. That was a tremendous shock for me.

What should I have done?

Suggestion: In retrospect, right from the hospital, I should have sought help proactively. What if he had a tongue tie that kept him from latching on and sucking properly? I don't think he had any, but what if I didn't have medical knowledge to know? What if my positioning during feeds was not proper? What if my expectations of what was normal were just wrong and ill-informed?

I should have sought help. I did, but in retrospect I can say not keenly enough. There are healthcare workers in a maternity ward ranging from midwives, all the way to lactation consultants who could give you help if sought. They offered help a couple of times, but in my opinion it did not seem keen or with a genuine effort from them. I also didn't know I could push for more. In the end, I felt very unsupported and unarmed with knowledge. This was in the setting of an African girl in a UK-based hospital.

What I would advise anyone going through the same is seek knowledge and ask questions proactively and with no shame, any and everything you need to know. What matters is that your baby is well catered for. Please ask for help, ask from the midwives, and if you feel like they're not able to solve the problem, ask politely if you can see a breast-feeding specialist, or whether they have any lactation consultants that could see you. Be proactive about speaking out and seeking help. Don't feel you would be disturbing them. That is what they are there for, but minority cultures in a foreign country must just know to be more proactive in speaking out. Persist too when you do speak out. Communicate your need and concerns effectively and persistently if required. Pray also that God sends you someone with empathy. A genuinely caring member of staff can make all the difference, so pray you find this.

> ***Pray also that God sends you someone with empathy. A genuinely caring member of staff***

can make all the difference,
so pray you find this.

I subsequently resorted to furiously pumping milk from my breasts after we couldn't master our latch properly. I attempted to pump every 3 hours, as advised following my research. He then got pumped precious breastmilk from a bottle. This was hard work, but the joy I felt made it worth it. I should have tried nipple shields (even though these can reduce your supply by preventing direct nipple stimulation. I explain this later on in the book). They may have helped me persist longer with trying to latch him on. My milk supply seemed low because it took me long hours to get the quantities I needed or wanted from pumping. Most times, a short while after pumping both breasts, I was due to pump again, according to the timing I used. I used the handheld madela pump, and this made my hands ache. It was also a single; so I had to do one side after the other. Ha-ha, oh my, the struggle! I must have some endurance; I think that's the only reason I could do that.

Noteworthy Lessons: The reason it reduced my supply was because of reduced stimulation of the nipples (direct stimulation of the nipples by the baby is many times more effective than stimulation from a pump). I often missed pumping sessions because of tiredness, and less frequent demand on the breasts also contributed.

I eventually researched what I could do to improve supply. I tried pumping at nights as this would increase my milk supply. It helped and my milk seemed to flow easily during the night, but this contributed to the sleeplessness. The need to get up from bed, go get the pump and bottles, or to wash and sterilise bottles in the middle of the night (which I often had to do to prepare for a next feed), the full alertness needed to sit up and pump each individual breast with a handheld pump at 3:00 am......! That was not a simple time.

Suggestion: If you're going through this pumping phase for whatever reason, in retrospect, I can tell you that getting a double pump which pumps both breasts at the same time will make your life easier. It would cut your pumping time in approximately half and catch milk loss from the unpumped breast while pumping one. Also, getting a pumping bra is something that might have helped me. This holds the pumps in place, leaving you free to do other things with your hands. It reduces the achy hands, and the stress associated with pumping. They may just cost you a little more money.

The following foods can help naturally improve your milk flow:

✦ Oats: High-fibre foods are thought to help improve the production of milk because of the beta-glucan content.

Beta-glucan is a compound that increases the secretion of prolactin in the body, and this is the milk-producing hormone. I generally eat a lot of oats when I have them. I love them for a quick, easy, and satisfying breakfast.

✦ Green leafy vegetables: These are part of a varied and healthy diet which is important for breastmilk production and nourishing your body, replacing what vitamins and minerals you lose into breastmilk secretion. Examples include pak choy (I grow these in my garden occasionally), broccoli, and kale. I tend to eat a lot of these.

✦ Ginger: I have always eaten a lot of ginger. My mum used it a lot in seasoning meats and you couldn't beat the taste of her seasoned meats. I use it the same way, in seasoning meat, and finely chopped and added to stir-fries. I have learned this helps to improve milk secretion.

✦ Fenugreek: I read about Fenugreek being good for improving milk secretion, and I tried the capsules. My milk quantity improved, but what followed was troubling flatulence that I couldn't bear. My son also seemed colicky and gassier after starting the capsules. I subsequently stopped them after realizing I was suffering the side effects, and the symptoms resolved on stopping.

✦ Last of all but most important, is drinking surplus amounts of water, as breastmilk is made up predominantly of water. This will help significantly.

This entire journey took me about 3months in total of breastfeeding, and then it gradually tailed off. He was having top up feeds with formula all this time. Since breastmilk was such a struggle to pump, I resorted gradually to more formula.

In writing this, I now recollect how I tried in my first journey because I often write the process off in my memory as though I did not try; and because of this, I've dealt with a lot of guilt for not trying, or not trying enough. It's something I would love to prevent anyone I can from facing; the guilt and regret. Those are very unpleasant feelings. Thankfully though, all of this led to the great learning I used for the subsequent journey, which made that a much more pleasurable and ecstatic experience, with highlighted lessons worth sharing. That subsequent experience, and the beauty of it, which often brought lots of tears (of joy) to me, lots of dancing moments, and a heart saturated often with gladness, is what compelled me to write all the lessons learnt, and to share it; hoping you too can experience like me, the beauty nature provides in the breastfeeding and infant nurture journey.

The next few chapters aim to arm you with the knowledge I wish I had the first time around. If you have tried but you absolutely cannot breastfeed your child in a circumstance I'd consider exceptional, then that's fine. You can give an alternative. Note that sometimes you may face some difficulty, but you can overcome it with help and support and you can still provide infant milk for your baby. I think it is important to understand just how key breastmilk is to the well-balanced development of your child's brain and their overall health; as having this knowledge alone can spur some people on to perseverance, which would enable them to overcome the challenges of breastfeeding. And don't forget, breastfeeding isn't just about giving breastmilk; but the very act of suckling a child on the nipple is itself important for the well-balanced development of your child.

Come with me further, let's see why.

The next few chapters aim to arm you with the knowledge I wish I had the first time around.

CHAPTER 2
BREAST MILK: JUST WHY IS IT SO IMPORTANT?

Why I chose it Personally

For me, the safety of knowing I was doing things the way the creator made them to be was simply enough reason to breastfeed. Even before finding out the details and having my eyes opened to the revelation of the purpose of breastmilk in a child's development, it satisfied me to know I was simply fulfilling purpose by breastfeeding. That is, doing what your breasts were meant to do. I can't explain it better than saying something in me craved the fulfilment that came with breastfeeding my child.

We can divide breastfeeding into these parts, which each have a unique benefit:

1. **Getting the child to have breastmilk, which shows all the benefits listed below.**

2. **The process and art of getting the child to suckle on the breast.**

3. **Feeding responsively and not on a scheduled basis.**

Suckling is a fundamental need for a child. One thing important to note is, whenever we miss out on nature's recommended ways, there is something we are depriving ourselves of which may not become apparent immediately. We often face the effects of not having these things, and we are usually neither able to realise the cause nor trace it back to its roots. From both suckling on the breast and responsively feeding or attending to a baby, they learn to trust. A man named David, who in his time was a writer, amongst many other things, put these words in his writings (between 1010-970 B.C),

"But You are He who took me out of the womb;
You made me trust while on my mother's
breasts." Psalms 22:9 NKJV.

Dating back to the ages, breastfeeding at the breasts has also had a fundamental role in building *trust, safety, security*, and much needed *comfort* into the developing psyche of a child. More on this later. But then, even more amazing is the realisation I came to of just how beneficial breast milk is. Mum K.I, a mum of three, and medical doctor with over a decades' experience working with kids, had this to say when asked about her mindset about breastfeeding and its importance before having her baby,

"Before the birth of my first baby, who had a fairly low birth weight, I had already decided that exclusive breastfeeding would help with adequate weight gain and boost her immunity. Over the past 14years of medical practice, I personally could attest to the effect of breastfeeding in the life of my paediatric patients. That helped me take a decision early, even before marriage, regarding breastfeeding. I also knew it would help with the bonding process and ease the colicky period."

I will start by summarising the components of breastmilk. According to this PubMed article, [PubMed is a scientific literature database offered to the public by the U.S. National Library of Medicine (NLM)]; Review of Infant Feeding: Key Features of Breast Milk and Infant Formula, Published online 2016 May 11,

"Mothers' own milk is considered to be the best source of infant nutrition. Extensive evidence has shown that breast milk contains a variety of bioactive agents that modify the function of the gastrointestinal tract and the immune system, as well as in brain development. Thus, breast milk is widely recognized as a biological fluid required for optimal infant growth and development. Recently, studies have further suggested that breast milk mitigates infant programming of late metabolic diseases, particularly protecting against obesity and type 2 diabetes.

Human breast milk contains carbohydrates, protein, fat, vitamins, minerals, digestive enzymes and hormones. In addition to these nutrients, it is rich in immune cells, including macrophages, stem cells, and numerous other bioactive molecules. Some of these bioactive molecules are protein-derived and lipid-derived, while others are protein-derived and indigestible, such as oligosaccharides. Human milk oligosaccharides (HMOs) possess anti-infective properties against pathogens in the infant gastrointestinal tract, such as Salmonella, Listeria, and Campylobacter, by flooding the infant gastrointestinal tract with decoys that bind the pathogens and keep them off the intestinal wall. Oligosaccharides also play a vital role in the development of a diverse and balanced microbiota, essential for appropriate innate and adaptive immune responses, and help colonize up to 90% of the infant biome.'

In summary, I say, human breast milk is nature's best targeted and designed feed for human babies. It protects their immune system by supplying immune cells to fight off initial exposure to the common pathogens in food, hence serving as a shield for the baby while he develops his own innate immune defences, and develops other systems, forming robust and well capable systems to handle all the microbes and toxins we inadvertently expose ourselves to in our environment. I believe breastfeeding is even especially more important as industrialisation continues to progress, and with it, the build-up toxicity in the environment, as the immune system needs to be stronger to withstand the challenges. We cannot compare the current toxic burden of our environment to what it used to be many, many years ago. This may be why I believe it is of utmost importance that we refocus our attention on breastfeeding and understanding just how vital it is for the normal functioning of a child. This will help us make better informed decisions to give them a good fighting chance for the environments they will grow up in. God will also make sure they are adequately equipped.

I believe breastfeeding is even especially more important as industrialisation continues to progress, and with it, the build-up toxicity in the environment, as the immune system needs to be stronger to withstand the challenges.

The Brain Development of your Child

One striking factor (amongst many others), that differentiates humanity from animals is our ability to think for ourselves. There are many other differentiating factors, but in my estimation, this is the most striking one. A Human's ability to create, to dominate a sphere, be judiciary over a matter, make laws and execute them, to rule; in summary, to carry out higher mental functions, differentiates us from all other creation. The resources breastmilk provides caters to the well-balanced development of these mental functions.

Nature tailors the human milk to the needs of the human infant, just like the milk of other mammals is tailored to meet the needs of their young. Humans have needs that differ from those of cows, some of which I have highlighted above. Cow babies have different needs. The milk provided for their young is designed by nature to cater to their most proficient use, for muscle mass, bulky growth, and brute strength. Cows traditionally were and still are in some parts of the world, used for farming due to the strength of their bulls (castrated males) and sheer muscle mass able to carry load and pull yokes along farmlands; creating the ridges and furrows used for planting. The bulls are also allowed to feed off the grain while treading it out. However, their use has shifted because of industrialisation and the replacement of animals with machines by farmers. The demand from consumers has also tailored how cows are bred to meet up with demands.

Can you see where I'm going with this? Milk produced from a human cannot, for instance, be used to feed a baby cow, or one might produce quite a lean but highly intellectual cow. Ha-ha! I doubt that, but hopefully you get the point. Human milk contains 1% protein and cow milk 3%. I often see humans consume high levels of concentrated protein for building muscle mass. From the distinction I made earlier, cow's milk contains more protein to cater to their specific need for muscle mass. Human milk, on the other hand, is tailored to developing higher mental functions to enable the human baby function at the capacity it was supposed to in this world. It enables development into a dynamic, resilient, and healthy baby, capable of change and adaptability. This is what breastmilk is purposed for.

The aim of this is not to put any shame or guilt on anyone. My aim is to clarify in our minds that there is a proper and unique distinction between components and functions performed by both milks. When this distinction is made and established in our minds, the emphasis I feel should then be on finding out how to make breastfeeding work best and to make it easy, so that many more people are able to get on without as many hindrances.

Preparation of your baby's gut for the world

The microbiome is the collection of the specific pattern of microorganisms (bugs) each person has lining their gut (intestines), and other parts of their body – the highest concentration being found in the gut. These microbes assist in several functions, including:

+ **Digestion of our food:** breaking down of more complex food particles we eat and releasing the more easily absorbable forms. For instance, according to this Harvard School of Public Health article titled 'The Microbiome', simple sugars are easily absorbed in the upper part of the small intestine, but more complex ones may travel on to the large intestine, and there the microbiota help to breakdown these compounds with their digestive enzymes. The fermentation of these hard to breakdown fibres by the microbes produces short-chain fatty acids (SCFA), and these SCFAs are noted to play an important role as a nutrient source, in muscle function and in prevention of certain chronic diseases. The article quotes a study by den Besten, Gijs., et al., called 'The role of short-chain fatty acids in the interplay between diet, gut microbiota, and host energy metabolism' and it found that these SCFAs may be useful in the treatment of ulcerative colitis, Crohn's disease, and antibiotic-associated diarrhoea.

+ *maintaining a healthy balance between the safe and the potential disease-causing organisms contained as part of the microbiome:* They keep this balance between the health-promoting organisms that are part of the microbiome, and those that can potentially cause disease, by competing with these potentially harmful bugs for nutrients and binding sites along the wall of your gut; keeping them from increasing in numbers unnecessarily and colonising and potentially invading our gut, causing disease. An example of this is what happens when a person who has had a long course of antibiotics develops clostridium difficile diarrhoea. Here, the antibiotic targeted at a certain bug or bugs also kills off the good bacteria in your gut, creating an imbalance between helpful and pathogenic bacteria and leading to a colonisation and invasion of the gut wall.

+ *mood and emotional regulation:* The brain-gut network plays an important role in our well-being, emotions, and ability to make intuitive decisions (as also noted by Dr Emeran Mayer in his research of the brain-gut networks).

+ *breakdown of the toxins we ingest in food:* which are increasingly unavoidable because of the progression of industrialization and its attendant increased toxic burden on the environment.

✦ *weight regulation, etc.*

The composition of our microbiome is determined by our DNA to start with, and then begins to be influenced and changed by dietary and environmental exposures right from birth. The diet from birth being either breast milk or formula; with each promoting a certain pattern of gut microbial composition, which is either health promoting or predisposing to disease. Environment from birth being whether we are born through the birth canal. The birth canal typically is the first place the child is seeded with the helpful microbes (found in the mother's vaginal lining) that eventually form part of their microbiota. Lactobacillus, for instance, is a microbe found in the mother's vagina lining that increases in quantity as the time of delivery nears. This bug is transferred to the baby during birth and plays an important role in helping the digestion of milk in the breast-fed baby. Skin-to-skin contact typically forms the next point of environmental contacts, and then other environmental exposures. For a child born via caesarean section, the first contact would be the skin of the mother.

Later on, other factors such as the diet we expose ourselves to – with certain patterns of diet promoting a more health preserving microbial composition than others, can either keep us well from disease or predispose the individual to certain diseases, and make them more vulnerable to environmental toxins. Also, whether or not we face other factors that cause an imbalance between the healthy and unhealthy microbes in our gut, such as prolonged antibiotic use – which kills off our good bacteria besides harmful bugs they're targeted at, e.t.c.

Professor Amy Brown, author of 'The Positive Breastfeeding Book' says,

> "We each have thousands of different species of bacteria, living in and on our bodies – in fact we have 10 times as many microbes as we have human cells. These microbes help breakdown the nutrients we eat, and eliminate environmental toxins that enter our bodies. You may have heard about 'good' bacteria affecting your digestive health, but more and more research is emerging that shows just how specifically important these bacteria may be. The types we have and don't have can affect everything from our mood, to our weight and our brain activity."

She goes on to say in her book,

> "Well a baby's very early experiences, how they are born, whether they get skin-to-skin contact with their mother, and then how they are fed – set up your baby's microbiome after birth. The milk they drink will make a difference to this. Breastmilk contains many different strands of good bacteria, which are introduced into your baby's digestive system. Breastmilk provides and encourages the growth of different bacteria than for-

mula milk. Breastfed babies have high levels of protective bacteria known as actinobacteria, while formula-fed babies have higher levels of pro-inflammatory bacteria called proteobacteria. This means that the microbiomes of breast and formula-fed babies are very different."

I discovered that altered microbiomes have been found in and linked with certain gut disorders such as irritable bowel syndrome and have even been linked to neurodegenerative disorders like Alzheimer's and Parkinson's disease. Dr Emeran Mayer also mentions this. I like to stress this area because it is very important; so here's some further information that might help explain things in my own language:

To summarise, once a baby is born, whatever forms its first exposure and introduction of its insides (i.e., gut lining) to the outside world in the form of food, goes a long way to determine how its gut microbiota is formed. This also ultimately greatly influences its capacity to handle foods and toxins in the environment. Breastmilk is the natural hypoallergenic feed for infants which provides a safe and non-toxic environment for this initial exposure to happen gradually, gently, quietly, and in safety. With breastmilk, gradual and controlled exposure of the baby's gut lining to the outside world and its potential pathogens (disease-causing organisms) takes place.

Continuing, breast milk bridges the gap between the baby's gut and the environment as it learns to handle food. Liken the impact of breastmilk to this saying I've coined, "Breastmilk helps to prepare the house." I believe this encapsulates the initial function of the maternal milk to some extent.

Take this example: an army needs to be trained in the safety of its camp before facing potential enemies from the outside. They don't start off in a war zone, or well they shouldn't. They should ideally be trained in the safety of their own camp, and then faced with an actual war situation when they have received enough training to help them defeat the enemy and come back alive. It would also be unfortunate to have a soldier trained by a commanding soldier who is ill-equipped to provide him with all the necessary training he needs on the battlefield.

Now, formula milk with all its components can be likened to the ill-equipped soldier, or to an 'artificial mothers' milk' not competent enough to prepare the baby's gut to face the outside world to the same extent that the mothers breast milk would. Breastmilk contains living tissue which changes with your baby's needs. It is considered 'intelligent milk' as it adapts to the needs of your baby.

Breastmilk contains living tissue which changes with your baby's needs. It is considered 'intelligent milk'

The experiences some babies have with first exposure to milk (other milk) can be likened to starting off in a war zone. The gut is immediately faced with things it must fight off, and components the body alerts to as 'foreign', even before the gut has a chance to be welcomed properly into this world. What's even more fascinating is the fact that these memories of our experiences on exposure to foods, known as gut experiences and gut memories, are stored away in the brains database, and influence how we relate to food, even our thinking and ability to trust to an extent. I know this must sound like a lot, but you do your research. This influences the child's receptivity to food. The child's first exposure to the world occurs at birth, and if this starts rockily, it teaches the baby subconsciously that the world or outside environment is unsafe to an extent, and could make them cautious, hesitant to an extent; with food and even people. All of this to an extent. Of course, many other factors also contribute to causing these personality developmental traits in a child, but this is just to point out aspects of breastmilk and infant feeding we don't often think of.

Infection-fighting properties

Human breast milk contains living antibody cells, and these are cells that help us fight off infection. These cells adapt and change as need be and are passed on from the mother's circulation onto the child's. Here is a breakdown of various anti-infective properties found in breastmilk which are not present in formula milk.

According to GP notebook, an online practise aid and learning resource for General Practitioners in the UK, with breastfeeding, there is:

✦ Reduced risk of gastro-intestinal infections, i.e., diarrhoeal illnesses.

✦ Reduced incidence of needing hospitalisation for respiratory tract infections in those babies breastfed – both a reduction in severity of viral and bacterial respiratory tract infections, and with a reduced risk of developing pneumonias as well.

✦ Reduced incidence of otitis media following colds, i.e., reduced occurrences of ear infections, as well as throat infections too.

✦ Necrotizing enterocolitis, a serious illness affecting small preterm babies in which the tissues of the intestines become inflamed and start to die, is less likely in breastfed babies.

Reduced rates of allergy with breast milk

You may have heard of cow's milk protein allergy. This is an array of allergic manifestations caused by proteins con-

tained in cow's milk which the body often recognises as foreign and which begins a chain of allergic reactions in some
children, showing effects in various systems like respiratory, digestive, skin, etc. They can often have diarrhoea type
symptoms, tummy upsets, are generally irritable and un-
happy babies, rarely settled and calm after feeding. They
may also have asthma-type chest symptoms, eczema skin
reactions, recurrent nappy rashes, etc. This, of course, is less
seen with breastfed babies who were exclusively breastfed
in early infancy.

There has been found to be a reduced risk of coeliac disease as well as irritable bowel disease, which are both auto-
immune diseases, in those breastfed as babies. Concerning
the increasing prevalence of allergy and allergic disorders
today, and its link to early diet and other factors in the environment, i.e., exposure to environmental toxicity, Maureen
Minchin, a historian, experienced lactation counsellor and
mother with vast amounts of research and publications on
the subject matter, who has also spent a majority of her life
campaigning on the return to the original paths for infant
feeding, and trying to show through her research how this
could reduce the epidemic of a host of dis-ease states we
experience today, says in her book titled 'Milk Matters',

"The Milk hypothesis asserts that the artificial feeding
of infants is the single greatest avoidable negative input into normal human development and health."

She says,

> "To me, western epidemics of allergy and autoimmune disease are the inevitable and predictable result of generations of infant dysnutrition, compounded by other environmental factors. Subtle as well as serious harms of artificial feeding echo and amplify through generations in unpredictable ways, due to both genetic and epigenetic influences."

She explains the harm caused by poor nutritional choices in early childhood – particularly choosing to formula feed instead of breastfeed, and how these have harmful effects on the child even down to the gene level, which means when they grow up, these can be passed on also to their children. Environmental factors we expose them to also play a role in determining health outcomes. The current toxic load in our environment really needs to be curbed. We can do our part by limiting exposure, both for ourselves and our children. This starts with identifying environmental threats – even as common as chemicals in our food e.g., pesticides, chemical fertilisers, and harsh preservatives, to the use of plastic in preserving our food where these are not coated with a food safe coating. Looking at safe and alternative ways to lead less disease creating lifestyles will preserve the lives of both us and our future generations, because we may tend to pass on these damages we acquire from the environment to them. Hence, even though the choice of infant feeding is not the only cause of disease states later and even early in life, it is a major cause and one that is often overlooked, and which can certainly easily be corrected.

Benefits for the child far into adulthood

From GP notebook, there is found to be a reduction in:

+ Obesity: 15% to 30% reduction in adolescent and adult obesity rates if any breastfeeding occurred in infancy compared with no breastfeeding.

+ Diabetes: Exclusive breastfeeding for at least 3 months – 30% reduction in the incidence of type 1 diabetes mellitus and a 40% reduction in type 2 diabetes mellitus.

+ Childhood leukaemia's and lymphomas: A reduction of 20% in the risk of acute lymphocytic leukaemia and 15% in the risk of acute myeloid leukaemia in infants breastfed for 6 months or longer.

+ Positive effects of breastfeeding on long-term neurodevelopment have been observed in preterm infants.

Other benefits I partook of

+ Fewer health challenges throughout infancy and into toddler years.

+ Economic benefits to the family.

✦ Easier feeding process, as I didn't have to make up bottles at night, or even during the day, and didn't have to get up from bed to go make up a feed, hence waking up totally and taking some time to get back to sleep, or never even being able to get back to sleep.

✦ Less hygiene issues as no worries about the contaminants in artificial milk or in poorly sterilized bottles.

✦ No issues of constipation because of erring in the mixing ratios of water to milk when reconstituting powdered formula milk.

✦ Less anxiety about running out of formula and needing to go find some in the stores urgently.

✦ No worries about having to preheat milk before feeding.

Benefits for your health: Reduced cancer risk

Breastfeeding is also said to give health benefits such as a reduced risk of ovarian and breast cancer in the woman. It helped me lose pregnancy weight, and even some pre-pregnancy weight! This is because of its high calorific demand on the human body. In the next chapters, I share more on how I dealt with this period of constantly feeling hungry. I also outline all of the life-changing lessons I learned on my journey and hopefully these will create greater ease for you in yours.

CHAPTER 3
SUCCESS, FINALLY

My second journey

Following my first breastfeeding experience and realising just how important breastmilk was, I was determined to make a change; and these changes guaranteed and eventually led to my success the second time around. I must admit that this is my experience, and I have done my best to include all aspects I saw played a part; so as not to give an incomplete picture of all the factors that helped me, because that would indeed be misleading. Please be patient with me if you hold different beliefs, as we can all still gain useful lessons from each other, even when our beliefs are different.

Mindset change, in my case, came from my deepening relationship with God. In this book, I have also referred to him as 'Creator'. For others, it could easily come from hearing more stories of people who have succeeded, or it could come from educating yourself on the subject via reading books on the subject just as an example. In my case, breastfeeding was something I really wanted to do. I expected there would be joy and beauty in it. I believed God had created me with the ability to breastfeed my child - He had made every woman, born a woman with breasts, with this innate ability, and if I wasn't confident my breasts could be up to the task, by this time I had learnt enough about the significance of my thoughts and words, and the power released from speaking the things we believe. So, I used this knowledge. I started to think, because I was realising more - God is so exceptional, and He is mindful when creating. He considers all of the little details. He does everything so intelligently and the systems He makes are always so sophisticated, as I had come to observe. My admiration peaked when one day I finally thought to myself, *Wow, He is a creative genius!* (If I could describe Him using those words).

I had suddenly come into a heightened awareness and an awakening; so to speak, of the fact that all of creation is truly excellent. In areas where I had let Him, I observed in my life how God had planned things so excellently, and indeed displayed great wisdom in His plans. And the realisation hit me that He created me too, and in fact, I had learnt that He refers to us humans as His 'masterpiece' creations. I was learning all of this from reading the Bible. Now, it might not seem to you that you are a masterpiece of the Creator, especially if, as a person, you often look down on yourself. As for me, I had always wondered, *is there more to this creation - me, us, than we currently know? Than we experience? Could it be that in different circumstances, there would be a lot more magnificent function and expression possible to humans than the current state of our world allows us to express and experience*? I then said to myself, "If I am so wonderfully made by a wise and intelligent Creator, then under the right or optimal circumstances, I expect my body to do amazing things - exactly what He planned originally for it to do." This, my friend, is the beginning of what inspired in me the confidence to try my body again – for breastfeeding.

My view of my body had changed. I started to view my body as a machine which had great potential. This informed the way I spoke about myself, and to myself. My words were more encouraging. I spoke with belief; not doubting my capacity. I spoke confidently about my body, and even to my body. I would say things like, "You're going to feed my baby and produce milk in surplus amounts for them." As you will see in subsequent parts of this book, this command actually cost me, but in the long run, speaking to my body was a good thing.

How an altered view of Self-love played a part

I also realised my body must need certain things like certain nutritious foods, to help it function at its best capacity and ability. I thought it must need rest also; to recuperate, cleaning and outside maintenance, as well as methods to check that what is going on inside is as it should be. These were all thoughts that had come to me. The desire to look after myself was now born out of a realisation of how amazing my body was, and just how amazing in function it might be if I gave it the right foods and the care it needed. Love filled my heart for my body, along with a desire to honour it. This is the definition of self-love I have learnt — one born out of love and the realisation of value. This kind of love requires that I would do also the things necessary to keep myself healthy, and not just whatever I feel like doing. It's self-love that comes with discipline as well. This was the beginning of my becoming health aware and piqued my interest in returning to the way the Creator originally planned for us to live; that we might live to fulfil the potential we all have deep down inside.

The winning outcome

Here, I will give a general overview of how my journey went with my second child, and in Chapter 4, I will give detailed insight into each challenge I overcame; how I did it and what I learnt from it, hoping it will add some knowledge for your own journey.

I would credit most of my success to the change in my mind-set and the determination I had to persevere through challenges. This time around, the difference in approach started from labour. I had learnt from my first child not to rush the onset of labour, but to let nature take its course. Your body will naturally expel the child when it's fully mature, all things being equal. Of course, there will always be abnormal situations where it is justified to help the body move along, so I can't make a blanket statement on this. However, where everything is in its normal functioning state, your body has its innate clock, which I like to call 'the auto-biology clock'; to highlight its automatic nature, which automatically and without prompt, performs its functions at their appropriate time. Look at menarche (the start of the menstrual cycle around puberty), menopause, the attainment of milestones in infancy, when teeth choose to erupt, when fontanelles (the soft spots on your child's head) close, etc.; these all happen on their own. The body recognises when it's time and prompts them to begin, with no need for external prodding. I feel like I must specify that these things happen as stated in the normal situations. I am not talking about the exceptions to the norm.

This leads me again to the lesson taken out from my initial experience where I felt like I'd waited too long for labour to start and tried to induce it myself by doing some of the rampantly recommended things – I walked, I climbed stairs, jogged on the spot, ate pineapples because of the bromelain content which is attested to help get things started down there.

Not anxiously trying to kick-start labour this time

Anxiety clouds judgement and can lead you to make poor choices. It heightens your perception of pain and limits your threshold for enduring things. Don't be anxious. Trust that you can do this. Your body can. It was created for this. The problem is in your mind and perception.

When my first child came out finally, well past the due date and when he was ready (and the delivery was seam-less), I remember feeling that he seemed so perfectly well adapted and ready for the outside world. I was particularly impressed with his reflexes and just how competent and robust they all seemed. He was just an excellent work of the Creator! I remember thinking just how perfectly sewn together all his parts were. I felt in retrospect that nature had its reason to take so long, and I made a mental note to wait in my future pregnancy and not anxiously try to rush the baby out. I remembered to apply these lessons in my second labour and this time, I had heard from God – He had spoken to me; promising that He would be with me through the delivery and safely deliver my baby. This is how God sometimes communicates with us. Thus, the second time around, I went into labour automatically, just a day before I was due. I had gone well past my due date with my first – as is often common with some first pregnancies.

Miraculous Pain Relief experienced in Labour

During the early phases of labour, before we got to the hospital, I felt the contractions come and go and was in pain with each contraction. We still had a lot of places to go before the hospital, to pick up my son from school, to the house to pick up some things, to drop him off with a family friend, and I wondered how I would bear the pain before we got to the hospital. I remember looking to God and asking Him for help with my pain relief. He simply asked me to keep my focus on heaven. I believe the aim was to keep my mind off the sensations of my pain, and instead focus on something that would release joy and peace to me. I pictured myself in the throne room in heaven, singing with the angels. As I imagined this, I sang out loud in the car that took me to the hospital. The pain would peak with each contraction, and that was the only time I felt it; at the peak. That my mind was elsewhere had somehow kept me from feeling the pain throughout the contractions. This made the pain bearable.

This was engaging the principle of focus and where we put it. The distraction in this case helped. You magnify the perception of your pain by focusing on it.

I must admit though, that it wasn't easy to focus on something apart from the pain and maintain that focus whilst the pain was screaming at you, but this is ultimately how we aim to live, where we can switch our focus, and maintain it on the real but unseen realm of the heavens. Here it takes a lot of intentionality. This activity seemed to somehow have the same effect nitrogen gas and air had on me, with me only feeling the pain at its peak. It was great. I thought I'd only document this experience in a book. I know not everyone accepts an experience like this, but I'm glad I do. Approaching God with child-like faith has opened me up to many supernatural experiences.

Benefits from obeying the midwife's instructions while in labour

Labour the second time was like my first, but faster; and I felt more in control because I used the lessons I had learnt from the first:

✦ Shout less. Instead of shouting, direct the energy into pushing. My mother said this to me during my first labour, when I had become preoccupied with expressing my agony with yells.

✦ To listen to the midwife and follow her instructions on when to push and when not to, despite the urges I felt.

This time, I felt more in control, so I could understand the processes going on in my body better. My midwife's instructions were a godsend during the pushing stage. She told me when to push and when to go against the urge to. She employed a very gradual method, gently teasing the head of the baby out of the introitus, just when she was about out; and by this was able to avoid any tearing I trusted in her instructions and controlled my urges, and this really paid off. The resulting delivery was that a bigger baby could pass without causing a tear. This, in itself was a miracle. God used this to teach me the difference between our works and His grace in enabling the accomplishment of a task. He likened His grace to the external conscious pushes, and our works to the internal rhythmic automatic muscular contractions that help to push the baby out towards the outlet. By themselves, these internal rhythmic and automatic contractions are often not powerful enough to fully deliver the baby; and if allowed to go much longer, they would cause a complete wearing out of the muscles of the womb by the time the baby was born. In this analogy, our efforts or human works are likened to the internal rhythmic contractions that try to push the baby out. Whereas His grace is the external push (in this case, from a force external to us) that, together with our efforts; propels us towards achieving our goals. I'll let the Holy Spirit explain this analogy further to you if you need it.

Round-the-clock breastfeeding within the first 48hrs

My baby began feeding immediately after birth, and I let her have her way. I was determined to let her feed on my breasts as long and as often as she wanted. She was content feeding on my breasts for the first 2days; I didn't worry she was hungry. She came on frequently, often falling asleep at the end of each feed. A newborn baby's stomach is only about the size of a walnut, and so they need to feed little and often. This is why they come on frequently to your breasts and seem hungry too often. It is not because you are not producing enough, contrary to what most newborn mums think.

By the end of the second day or so, I was engorged. My breasts felt fuller. She was swallowing more when feeding - my milk had 'come in'. I attribute the earlier 'coming in' this time around, to the frequency with which I was putting her to the breast (which was as frequently as she demanded) in those first 48hrs. It signalled my brain that the demand was higher, and it produced sooner. My milk came in later with my first, and I attribute this to the fact that I often bottle-fed in those two days and only put him to breastfeed occasionally, as we had trouble getting a good latch. This put less demand on my body to produce milk and sooner.

Picture each attempt to feed your baby from the breast within those first few days, as 'withdrawals' taken from your body. Now picture that your brain assesses how many 'withdrawals' are made over the first 24-hour period and notes this. It also then notes how many withdrawals are made over the second 24-hour period, averages the two and then gives you output based on this. It follows then that every demand made by your baby must be put through to your breasts and hence to your brain; as this is your body's way of 'registering' the demand. Doing this and letting your body recalculate the demand as it comes should solve all forms of supply issues.

The following things interfere with an accurate calculation of demand by your body:

+ Using breast pumps registers as demand (although less effective than direct suckling) and hence increases supply. If the combination of your direct suckling, and pumping, are in excess of what the baby needs, this can lead to oversupply issues.

+ Using nipple shields (the reduced direct suckle registers as reduced demand and hence reduced supply follows).

✦ Mechanical stimulation of the nipples (in expressing) registers as demand and leads to supply.

Now, these might be useful to produce temporary relief when you are engorged or hurting, but might also lead to an increase in supply in the long run if continued besides direct and regular suckling from the nipples.

The challenges of the first few weeks

I developed excoriations with fissures around the nipple and was engorged. All these issues subsequently resolved as my supply regularised, and my nipples got used to feeding frequently after the first few weeks. But at the beginning, after a few days of breastfeeding, my nipples had started to hurt; I cried, wailed, and wanted to give up a couple of times. The crying was both from the pain of breastfeeding on nipples with wounds, the internal pain from the pressure of engorged breasts, and sleeplessness. There was also the issue of dehydration. I realized I hadn't been drinking enough water. You need to drink more when breastfeeding. Remember, this was the first time I had experienced breastfeeding in this capacity. For my first journey, formula helped do some shifts while I fed from my breast on a few shifts and mostly pumped. It had become painful enough to make me dread oncoming feeds. I would experience anxiety and hesitance while I tried to latch her onto my sore nipples. I would cry, wait, and then take a deep breath and put my nipples into her mouth. She had a strong suck, with a powerful pull; I would often feel the tug of her suckling deep within my breasts. This was as dramatic and difficult period, but thankfully it only lasted a few weeks. Our breastfeeding journey lasted well over a year, compared to this initial painful period, and I am thankful for it.

Then there was the initial oversupply because of my words. I had constantly asked for this, because I was so determined to breastfeed, and I wanted my baby to have surplus and lack for nothing. I wanted to throw her a lavish breast-milk party, but I didn't know it didn't work like that for the breasts producing the milk. Where would the excess be stored? This produced the engorgement. Engorged means, 'overfilled with fluid'. It constantly engorged my breasts for the first approximately two weeks — hard, rock solid, and massively enlarged.

✦ Pumping to relieve the pressure didn't seem to help, and I later learnt if I continued it would rather increase my supply further, as I was also fully breastfeeding.

✦ I was never efficient with self-hand expression, and definitely not to any capacity sufficient to provide relief from the pressure I felt inside.

✦ Going in the warm shower and 'letting it drain' didn't work. It felt for me like letting out only a few drops of fluid from a backed-up and clogged-up pipe. In fact, I would even get further let-downs of milk while in the shower and the pain from further expansion was not enjoyable.

Healthcare staff advised these things, so they must work for some people to bring relief during these emergency times. Some of these things might work for you to cause relief during this time, but none did for me. I share in chapter five what worked for me under the heading 'Dealing with Engorgement and Blocked Ducts'. In the end, one important factor in my journey was a willingness to persevere through all difficulties and to hold out for success in the end.

Through regularly feeding her as she desired and hoping she would drain my breasts on each feed to provide relief, things eventually regularised. I, of course, had repented and was urging my body by my words to regularise its milk supply. My body recognised the amount of milk she was demanding and accurately calculated this because there was no interference from other expressing activities, and eventually self-adjusted supply to correct the oversupply issue. There was a lot more I suffered, and many more real-life lessons I learnt from the journey. See in chapter 4, where I delve in detail into this period - the initially gory and then subsequent light and fun-filled journey of my second breastfeeding travel. But before we get into that, I want to show you Maureen Minchin's experience as she shares in her book titled 'Milk Matters'. Maureen Minchin is a medical historian, an experienced lactation consultant, and a mother. Her words really resonated with me, as she seems to have had a similar personal experience as me:

> "I was 'an elderly primip' in the 1970s, bombarded with free formula samples from the hospital and clinic, having my children comp-fed without my consent. I suffered the agonies of the damned during my first three tortured months of breastfeeding with hospital-induced nipple fissures, until reading Dr Mavis Gunther's Infant feeding, and healing those 'cracks' in two days. (I cheered to read that Mavis thought 'cracks' 'a slovenly term used only by those who have not troubled to see what the injury is).'

> Thanks to my mother, my son, my research background and Mavis Gunther, I learned how to breastfeed pain-free and joyfully – no thanks to either multiple medical personnel consulted, or timid self-help groups unwilling to offend doctors by giving 'medical' advice. In fact, had my mother not empathised with my pain in those first three months, and assured me that 'When it gets better, it is marvellous, there's nothing like it,' I would have joined all my educated middle-class friends of middle-class mothers, who had moved on to bottle-feeding. (Instead I evolved into a long-term breastfeeder, lactating for the best part of ten years with my three children. For which I am grateful as I approach seventy without osteoporosis or reproductive cancers!) So I feel nothing but empathy for those who experience the agony without the needed support and

solutions. Been there, know it's hideous, but also know that women can survive it, and that doing so is worth the effort it takes."

Despite the difficulties of breastfeeding, when you move past this stage, it blossoms into such a beautiful and deeply satisfying experience for both mother and child. It is very deeply fulfilling too. So, if perseverance through the initial phase is one of the challenges you face, know that the latter outcome is worth persevering for.

Despite the difficulties of breastfeeding, when you move past this stage, it blossoms into such a beautiful and deeply satisfying experience for both mother and child. It is very deeply fulfilling too. So, if perseverance through the initial phase is one of the challenges you face, know that the latter outcome is worth persevering for.

CHAPTER 4
ALL THAT I LEARNED

I asked one mum what support she would have liked to have on her breastfeeding journey, and she had this to say:

> *"I wish they had outlined all that can go wrong,*
> *and the fact that some women may not be*
> *able to breastfeed properly on the first day*
> *due to not having enough milk. If I had a pre-*
> *understanding of all different scenarios that*
> *could play out, my mind could be*
> *at rest and less worried"*
> *- Mum T.I.*

In this chapter, I have outlined every lesson from my breast-feeding journey.

The Breastfeeding Process

This is a brief overview of the hormonal processes taking place as you breastfeed. With every feed, as the baby latches on to your nipple and begins to suckle, he stimulates the sensitive nerve endings on your areola (the area of darkened skin around your nipple with bumps) which are called Montgomery's tubercles. These nerve fibres transmit the message to your brain, saying it's time to let down milk for the baby who's calling at the breast. Your brain then releases a prolactin-releasing hormone, which instructs the responsible cells to release more prolactin. When this is released, it stimulates the milk to be produced by your glands. Oxytocin causes milk let-down into your breasts, which then serve as the storage tank from which the milk can be let out into your baby's mouth.

Oxytocin is also the feel-good hormone and promotes bonding with your child. Oxytocin is also responsible for the discomfort you may feel in your lower abdomen when feeding. It does this by causing contractions of your womb whenever you feed, to help the involution or shrinkage process. This pain can be relieved by taking mild analgesics where needed. This all happens rather quickly when you breastfeed. Your body was made to do this. This comes naturally. I'm trying to get you to see the capacity of your body, so you may believe you can do this. I am doing this because

I have found out that what we believe greatly impacts the outcome we see.

Power in Your Tongue

A very important role was played by my words, and what I spoke stemmed from what I believed. Because my perspective of my body had changed, I addressed myself with hope and confidence in the fact that I would be able to breastfeed sufficiently.

See how I changed: My mindset had always been one of worry about whether I could breastfeed. I, for some reason, lacked trust in my mammary glands' ability to produce for me. Some of you may share this concern.

Next, I seemed to have more faith in one breast's ability to produce, than in the other. I notice this is a concern shared by others too. As I grew in mind change, I noticed how very demeaning and detrimental it is to your body's eventual productivity, when you lose faith and trust in its ability to do what it was meant for. Just like humans, our bodies also tend to live up to what we think of them. The concern about our bodies failing us is one that seems to be shared by many.

I changed to speaking confidently about my body as I began to realize the great capacity it was created with, and that it was created by a perfect God. I also spoke to my body; as in a normal conversation, telling it all the things it would do. I asked for an oversupply, and I later realized this was wrong. I thought I would be catering abundantly to the needs of my child, but didn't think about the storage capacity of my breasts. So, I suffered with terrible engorgement in the first few weeks. Of course, I repented and began asking for my supply to be regularised to suit just what we needed. I must confess here that in my case, this ability to speak and see the things I say come through comes from knowledge of my privileges as a child of God and not something else. My words had come true to an exactitude of my eager confessions. It is very important to first believe what you're saying, and to be consistent in this. Your body responds to words spoken out of your belief.

Vision, Doggedness, Perseverance: A Mindset

I had a vision in my mind of success with breastfeeding and believed bonding would be such a beautiful experience. This vision kept me going, and because I knew it was very achievable, I had no justification in my mind to cut the journey short and put away my dream. Hence, despite all the challenges I went through, that would have been more than enough reason to quit, quitting was just not an option. I had considered buying formula bottles a couple of times when the journey was tough; those late nights struggling both with sleeplessness and the constant demand on my boobs. My nipples were sore, but despite this, I realised introducing formula would be counterproductive. If you want your milk supply to be established and sufficient, then using formula is counterproductive. This is because it establishes lesser demand from your body, which in turn communicates to your brain that the child is requiring less milk, as your brain does not register the actual demand of your child who is being satisfied by formula, and so your body reduces its supply. This can then result in an inability to eliminate formula later on.

The clear principle is this: You want your body to register just how much milk your child desires. And this can only be achieved if you put your child to the breast whenever he wants to suckle. As such, reducing this demand by using decoys like dummies, or proper supplementing with formula, may eventually lead to a reduced supply. Beware of cluster feeding periods and the use of a dummy during this time.

All these explained difficulties one may encounter, eases off after the first few weeks for the majority, and breastfeeding becomes almost reflex; a skill learned. So, you mostly just need to hang on for the initial phase and then it becomes a lot easier as you get used to it, and your nipples stop hurting.

Providing fuel for your machine: Why am I so hungry all the time? Hydration and a nutritious diet

Breastfeeding is an intensive metabolic process, and it demands a lot of energy or fuel from your body. That fuel needs to be replaced and provided for by your diet. Also, because breast milk is made up to a large extent by water, your water intake should be optimal. Thirst and your urine colour are good ways to measure your hydration. Normally, your urine should be a pale amber colour and become more orangey the less hydrated you are; i.e., the more hydrated, the paler your urine, the less hydrated, the darker. I noticed a clear correlation between how much water I was taking and how well I was lactating. My let-down was often almost instantaneous when I was well hydrated, and milk flowed easily. When I knew I hadn't been drinking enough water, my milk would take a bit longer to come. Baby would have to suckle a lot more, and it would also seem to take a lot longer for them to get filled on the breast. Some people can erroneously assess this as not having enough milk, when in reality, all they need is sufficient water.

I felt hungry often, and sometimes even just after eating. This is because of the increased energy demands on your body, and your body craving high energy foods. When I didn't meet these demands, I lost weight. Now, this got me back to my pre-baby weight which I liked, but you should also supply the energy demands of your body during this time. In retrospect, I should have eaten a lot more, knowing that the increased hunger and appetite was because of the increased demand. I struggled with this because I wasn't clear on how much to feed myself due to never seeming satisfied. In healthy adults, your appetite or hunger should be a trustworthy indicator of when you need to eat. If you haven't had problems regulating your appetite before, please eat to satisfy your appetite/hunger. Trust your body to appropriately signal its needs and feed it to meet the demands. That would be my perspective.

Start the bonding early and immediately; Imprint on your baby

Consider this: your baby is an expected guest coming into the world. How would you welcome a guest coming into your country for the first time, assuming they were to be hosted at your house? Especially if you wanted to ensure them a soft landing, prevent culture shock, and help them form a good impression of the environment from their first exposure? I'd suggest you'd welcome them at the airport, make them feel honoured and somewhat important, ease them of their burdens - by taking their bags/coats, help them relax and rest, etc. Now, just to paint a picture: Would you offer them food? The most representative of your culture, and one they're most likely to appreciate? I certainly would. So, imagine if they were to have bad diarrhoea and tummy upset for days with the first meal they had from your hosting, or within the first few days of their arrival in your home/country. I believe that would definitely form a lasting impression and may affect for a long time how they respond to food offered in a new country/place. This is because humans have a memory that stores such gut experiences and affects our later responses; even without our knowing, as we use these memories when weighing new decisions. This happens.

Now bring this back to a child entering the world for the first time. To help start the formation of your child's psychological outlook on this world, you want to give them the warmest welcome possible. If the start off is not as good, maybe because of illness, difficult delivery, or them needing to be taken away to the newborn unit, that's beyond your control and an impression can still be repaired when you later start your bonding process.

Take mummy D's story, for example, she says,

"I had a Caesarian section and my son had to be taken away to the NICU immediately. We were apart for a while; a nurse brought a syringe for me to attempt to extract breastmilk after I left the theatre... I only got about a teardrop portion, then we started thinking we would need formula. I thought the teardrop volume

was inconsequential but the nurse thought otherwise. She took the syringe away to administer to him in NICU. Later on that day, I was wheeled to the NICU and asked to put him to breast... Turned out I didn't need formula."
- Mum D. A.

Otherwise, in normal circumstances, be there to give them an initial warm embrace. Give skin to skin for enough time to calm and reassure them. This regularises and settles both their heart rhythm and the pace. Offer them food (breast-milk) after some skin to skin, then continue the bonding as soon as possible (after they have been cleaned off and handed back to you by the nursing staff). *The goal is to form a first good impression, and this, like the name implies, should be the 'first' impression, so it matters what happens in those first few hours after birth.* We want to make them feel welcome. Offering food matters too because breastmilk is the calmest, most gentle introduction to the world you could give a child. It also contains all the human soldiers that help organise and stand guard in their guts.

The goal is to form a first good impression, and this, like the name implies, should be the 'first' impression, so it matters what happens in those first few hours after birth. We want to make them feel welcome.

Apart from the obvious external environment: air, water, skin, clothes, etc., the next place their bodies come into contact with the environment is their gut, and so you want a trusted, safe, and gentle exposure to this fresh and un-prepared gut. Your breastmilk is the safest, most gentle, and most reliable preparation that could provide this. Your milk gradually introduces them to the world, while your embrace comforts, reassures and protects them; making them feel safe and cared for in the new environment. They can then feel safe to sleep. And this gradually eases their experience into the world.

Be proactive in seeking support; including partner support

Of the mums questioned in the course of my writing, one mum felt that she received adequate support from her partner, and this helped her cope better on her journey. She shares,

> *"He had perfect understanding of the challenges I faced and was often there to sit with me and talk through the sleepless nights where I had to stay up breastfeeding. He understood he couldn't help me feed, as our child would not take a bottle, but his being there to keep me company, his showing support, and encouraging me to rest when he saw I needed to since I was the only one who could*

feed the baby, was all the support I needed."
- Mum T.K.

Also highlighting the need for partner support, another mum had this to say when asked if she thought her spouse understood the challenges women face during their breast-feeding journeys,

"Yes, my spouse understood the breastfeeding journey and the associated challenges mainly because I spoke out, expressed myself and got him involved."
- Mum K.A.

I recommend that as a gift you get your spouse a book explaining what a dad should expect in pregnancy, and postpartum; including preparing for breastfeeding and getting ready to be a support. A couple of titles are available on Amazon. Mum K.A. had this to say when asked about the support she eventually got.

"My husband was my support base. He made my journey easier, I must say. We were far away from any close family, so natural instinct played its role amongst us. He would help with meals when I couldn't, to keep up with the milk flow. While breastfeeding, at times, I could get some help from him with breast pumping from the other boob. Emotional connections with some physical touches from our spouses can help alleviate post-natal stresses and help with

breastmilk flow. I could take some sleep while he helped out with feeding the baby. We had lots of stored up milk from pumping. In order to ensure we both didn't get burnt out, we took turns especially during the colicky period to keep awake and stay with the child."

In these first few days, you will most likely need someone to show you or check that your baby is latching on well, and you may have questions about what to expect, what's normal, what's not normal, or whether all is well with your feeding. Proactively seek support. The hospital has well-trained staff specifically stationed to provide support to breastfeeding mothers, so use the service if you need any help at all. Be proactive in seeking this help and in asking questions. I would advise you get all your questions answered as soon as is possible. Take a note of the numbers to call and keep in contact with them even when you go home. Call them whenever it is necessary. Don't feel like your concern is too little, or like you'd be bothering them unnecessarily. They are there to give you this help, so feel comfortable in requesting the service.

This was something I improved on with my second pregnancy and asking for support made an enormous difference in the outcome for me. I've detailed the input I got under subsequent headings. A mum interviewed during my writing said this about her own experience:

"With my second child, my breasts were engorged. I suffered from mastitis and very sore nipples. They had somehow managed to miss a tongue tie in my baby."
- Mum I. D

In her case, it was eventually discovered that her baby had a tongue tie, but not before she'd gone through a great deal with the poor latch.

You can get the midwives to check if your latch is good. Tongue tie can be a reason for poor latch and it is not any fault of yours. If you're concerned about this, you can get someone to assess for this, and if they don't know or can't assess, they should point you in the direction of someone who can. You can get the midwives to check if your bleeding is normal. Ask about tummy aches/pains if any, ask about the colour of baby's poos, the frequency of wet and dirty nappies, how often to give him a bath, what skin care lotions/oils or cream to use, nappies/wipes, anything!

Actually, my midwife gave me the best advice on what to use in cleaning baby's bum and this was the most hypoallergenic option. So be free to ask all of the questions you need to ask. Be okay with not having information and then seek the answers. Be a good student. In the end, if it helps your baby, it would have been worth all the effort.

I do not intend to list the baby products I used specifically for my baby, as that will be out of the scope of this book. You can easily also find out this information from those around you who have had babies and see what they recommend. But as always, you will have to make your own decisions on what to use on your own baby. It's always an intuitive thing, with some research. I personally watched and read through best baby product reviews and saw the commonly or uniformly mentioned products and then went for those. It was pricey, although to our benefit. We ended up barely getting anything at all for my second pregnancy, as we still had things from the first pregnancy in great condition, and knew enough to avoid excessive buying. But it's hard to know the first time around all that you'll need, and what you won't end up using, so buy what you think you'll need & can afford. It is possible to raise a healthy and very happy child on minimum budgets.

Latching

Letting the baby latch or attempt to latch on to the nipple is recommended as the original design. They will often need your support to guide them to a position that's safe for both of you. I learnt its best to place your nipple directly over her upper lip, with the nipple pointed at her nostrils, then gently slide down into her wide opened mouth, so the nipple points towards her palate, i.e., the roof of her mouth.

Placing the nipple over their upper lip gets them to open their mouths wide for you. If you feel they don't have it open wide enough, try again until it is, but don't wait too long until the baby is exasperated. It's best to try to latch with everyone calm.

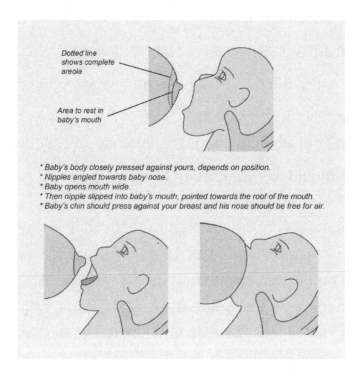

Dotted line shows complete areola

Area to rest in baby's mouth

* Baby's body closely pressed against yours, depends on position.
* Nipples angled towards baby nose.
* Baby opens mouth wide.
* Then nipple slipped into baby's mouth, pointed towards the roof of the mouth.
* Baby's chin should press against your breast and his nose should be free for air.

Checks for correct latch:

✦ With the correct latch, you aim to point the nipple towards the roof of your baby's mouth and get more of the breast inferior to your nipple into their mouths.

✦ When properly positioned and latched, your breast should ideally not press against or cover airflow into her nostrils.

✦ Their chin should also be apposed to the lower segment of your breasts when positioned correctly and latched properly.

✦ There should be suckling and swallowing.

✦ The baby should be more settled when coming off the breast, indicating a good feed.

✦ Pain or discomfort should be minimal and endurable.

✦ You should feel your breasts empty.

The tongue is very important for the suckling function, and when correctly latched, a good portion of the breast inferior to your nipple (inferior areola) should lie over their tongue, and when they suckle, the squeezing motions help rhythmically direct milk flow down your ducts and into their mouths. The centre of the pressure, is then on the areola, muscles surrounding the ducts, and the ducts themselves. When incorrectly latched, a good portion of the pressure is centred around your nipple and skin, along with the ridges of the hard palate grazing against them. This causes breakages and irritation. This can be traumatic and discourages many people from breastfeeding.

It is important to note that a virgin nipple, not accustomed to that degree of intense and regular stimulation (as would be the case with most people), will face a normal level of discomfort initially, before eventually adapting to the new level of activity. This may occur by an adaptation of the skin surrounding the nipple to its new level of activity.

How do I know a 'normal' level of discomfort?

Discomfort here differs from pain. Painful breastfeeding is not sustainable – you will either cut the journey short or lose your sanity. With what I call a 'normal' level of discomfort, it will of course not feel pleasurable; mostly because it is new, but it should be endurable. You should be able to see this activity as sustainable. You should also not notice obvious harm to your nipples or the skin around your nipples, and you should not have to feel damned or shed tears before feeding your baby. If a latch feels intensely uncomfortable, or painful, take it out and try again.

Should I endure a painful latch to let the baby feed?

Your desire to let your baby feed, and feed enough, might outweigh your immediate concern for yourself and your nipples, as can be with a concerned mother, but in the long-term, for breastfeeding to be sustainable for all the months you will need to feed, and even years for some people, 'slow and steady' will see you through. Starting with a lot of enthusiasm and giving your all, and often 'enduring' through painful and wrong techniques, will see you to exhaustion and eventually, the brink of dropping it all. Do not feed on a painful latch, only because this usually means that you are positioned incorrectly, or she is not properly latched on. And continuing a painful latch with the mindset to 'endure it' to feed your baby, will mean more painful feeds in the future.

Your baby will need to feed again not too long from now, and she will need to latch on again, and then you stand to face the added pain of a new latch on a sore nipple. Sequential repetitive improper latches accumulate micro trauma to the skin around the nipple and will eventually lead to broken skin if not stopped. By enduring, I got to this point unfortunately.

How to withdraw from an incorrect latch

It can be difficult to withdraw your nipple after the baby has latched on hungrily. The best way I found to do this was to slide a clean index finger between the gums of the baby, gently separating their gums wide enough to create a safe space to withdraw my nipple.

Responsive nurture – Attending to the baby's call for help

A child cries, it hears its mother or father or beloved adult responding to its cries, and it says "My cry is having an effect on them, but they're not picking me up; even though I know they're responding. That means they can't help me for some reason, but I can still trust them," versus "I cry and I can see them there or I know they're there, but they're not responding at all to my cries. It has no effect. It's either I can't trust my ability to cry out for help as effective, or I can't trust and depend on them to respond to my need." This sows a seed of insecurity in the developing child's psyche. Insecurity is followed closely by detachment from the caregiver and a sense of independence prematurely. Walls begin to go up in the developing child's heart. This forms the very start of their worldview.

When I cried out in pain during one of my breastfeeding sessions, I had just said as I came to the end of my withholding, "Well, if I perish, I perish" and then holding my injured nipple close to the mouth of my hungry daughter, I put the raw nipple into her mouth trying to escape as much of an improper latch as I could. I won't describe the pain I felt, but as I sat there in between tears and sobs, I finally cried out in frustration to God. I asked him why he made it so hard; I asked what this difficulty benefitted us. I asked why something simple and essential had to be so difficult. Then something special happened - I heard and saw Jesus, with my 'inner eye' (This just means spiritual sight, and is available to Christians). He was sobbing alongside me, and explained "it wasn't meant to be like this... but the fall of the man and all of creation has had far-reaching effects, even much more than many imagine." Merely seeing in that moment that He shared my pain, and was as concerned about it, was so healing for me. Even if that did not take away my pain that night, His responsive nature reassured me His heart was with me and He could be trusted. In the same way, a child is reassured when it sees or hears its caregiver responding to its cries for help, even if they can't solve the problem immediately.

> *The fall of the man and all of creation has had far-reaching effects, even much more than many imagine.*

I'm not saying adopt a slave type pressure on yourself to do this every time and begin to feel guilty if you don't. I'm simply sharing with you the heart posture that children need to be raised with. A simple sharing of this perspective and having this understanding will drastically improve things in the way you relate with your child and this change will happen even unconsciously to you. The change has to start from our minds first.

Responsive breastfeeding

Responsive breastfeeding or breastfeeding on demand is the best way. It is natural. Humans are created to know when it's time to eat. The body was well made and can alert a person to when it's time to take in some more food for fuel or nourishment. A baby communicates this need for food by crying, or rooting, which is where he or she starts to move their mouths around in the direction where they anticipate the nipple would be.

By observing your child for even a few moments, you can pick up the signs or cues for when she's ready to feed. Feed her as soon as you notice this. It should also be convenient for you.

Attending to a baby's needs on cue, and consistently, is also how they learn to trust. They learn security, and this is very important for how they develop into adult later in life. A lot of the insecurity deeply ingrained in our minds and thought processes starts with how we were treated in early childhood. Having the baby's needs met in a consistent and prompt manner, teaches her developing mind the world is a safe place. It shows her she is in caring hands and teaches her she can trust this individual to care for her. It brings a sense of security into her psychological development. This sense of security helps form her brain and her earliest thought processes, giving her the right foundation. She starts off relationships with other people in a healthy way and with a healthy perspective.

A lot of the insecurity deeply ingrained in our minds and thought processes starts with how we were treated in early childhood.

I was taught by the Holy Spirit never to let my baby cry and see me being unresponsive to her crying (as much as possible), and to try to communicate with her by talking when I'm unable to get to her but in proximity, e.g., when driving and she's crying in the back seat. In these cases, I would simply speak to her and try to explain we were going home, and I couldn't get to her now. It didn't stop her from crying all the time, but it communicated responsiveness and it let her know her communication was being heard and acknowledged, and that I might not have been able to reach her but was responding to her cues and trying to explain something. In her mind, this would give her an idea that there was something different happening this time; why I wasn't able to reach her, and then she could learn that maybe when she was riding in the back seat, in that scenario, mummy wouldn't be able to reach her for some reason. This is how babies and children learn about our world. We create routines they learn to depend on through our consistent actions and patterns, and routines give them structure, which is something they can lean on as it shapes both their behaviour and what they come to expect from their new world.

How do I know the baby is getting enough milk with each feed?

+ You see suckles and hear swallows.

+ They have sufficient wet and dirty nappies per 24-hour period.

+ They are gaining weight appropriately.

+ They seem settled after each feed, although they may occasionally be unsettled for reasons other than their satiety.

+ You can't overfeed a breastfed baby. They demand just as much as they want and are free to unlatch when they feel full. It's also more difficult to force feed a breast-fed baby. On the other hand, bottle feeding makes for easier overfeeding, or even underfeeding; due to fixed/ less flexible adjustment of feeds.

With breastfeeding, the baby determines how much they eat – as much or as little, until they're satisfied, and to meet the need for the phase of growth. Bottle feeding requires that you follow a prescribed schedule for feeds, but what if your child wants more than the quantity prescribed? Wants more of milk at one time than the other? What do you do when they don't want to finish the last ounce? If it was in your breast, it wouldn't go to waste. You wouldn't be tempted to force them to finish it. Do you make them finish the bottle to complete a feed or does their appetite determine when they've completed the feed?

Breastmilk as a pacifier

I found that breastmilk sorted most of her problems, and at times when she would cry for no understood cause, I found breastfeeding her seemed to settle it all. One night, I had woken up to feed her and she continued to cry. It was within our first 2 months. I did all I thought needed to be done – I had checked her nappy, rocked her, checked the room temperature to make sure she wasn't too hot or cold, made sure she was clean (I often found keeping her skin clean, as in giving her a bath or a rinse with water, solved most of her problems too), but this night, she continued to cry and did so despite my rocking. She had recently breastfed and didn't seem hungry. Now, having to walk back and forth and rock a child to sleep when you yourself are sleepy is one of the hardest things I faced in early postpartum. So, on this one night, while amid this episode which sometimes occurred for us, I had a thought: to put her to the breast whenever she was discomforted, as it would bring her comfort, no matter what the problem was. I did this, and she stopped crying, and subsequently slept off. After this, whenever she was discomforted and I had checked through the reasons listed above, I'd just put her to the breast, and it always calmed her down. I've come to recognise these thoughts as coming from God. They're His way of helping me with light (knowledge) when I feel I'm in darkness (ignorance/confusion).

> *I've come to recognise these thoughts as coming from God. They're His way of helping me with light (knowledge) when I feel I'm in darkness (ignorance/confusion).*

Adequate comfort from breastmilk during illnesses and supply of immunity

Breast milk came in handy the few times when my baby was ill and irritable from either teething, or she had got a tummy bug from somewhere. The illnesses happened few and far between, but when we found ourselves fighting against a tummy bug (in those moments where she didn't want anything to eat), I found breastmilk most soothing for her. She would only accept breastfeeding and tended to spend most of her time there. Recovery seemed quicker, and she was back to herself in almost no time, actively playing and laughing again, even if still recovering.

It is useful to know that for a bug you the mum have also been exposed to, your breastmilk at that time of illness can help provide targeted immunity to help combat the infection for the child. What happens is this: When you are exposed to a bug, as is often the case in whole family exposure, you may not be ill with it. In fact, you may have no symptoms at all, but your body produces immune fighter cells to attack and kill the bug. Your body also passes these fighter cells onto the baby in breastmilk to help them fight off the bug, since it anticipates they may have also been exposed. Formula, on the other hand, cannot contain immune cells and is not comparable to breastmilk, which is a living tissue. A tissue is made up of active cells, and that is what breastmilk qualifies to be called because of its active cell content. According to this GP notebook article titled 'Breast Milk',

> "Human breast milk includes secretory IgA, lactoferrin, peroxidases and lysozymes. These proteins are partly to protect the baby from infection. IgA forms a barrier in the baby's gut to protect against invading bacteria. Lactoferrin serves to deprive any invading bacteria of iron, and peroxidases and lysozymes both have an anti-bacterial action."

Breast milk also 'grows with the child' – it is basically mother nature in milk form, mothering the child and tending to its needs as they come up, modifying along with the child's needs. We can see formula as a 'foster parent' which doesn't have the innate capacity within it to mother a human child effectively since it is not of the same species. Formula is milk made from cows and modified to feed human babies. Some formula are made from soy, so they're plant based and not from cows. Goat milk formula is a newer milk also in circulation, but they're basically all milk obtained from animal parents, originally made for their animal babies. And while these have come in handy over the years and solved many problems for lots of people, nothing can beat human milk from a human parent for its own baby.

Breastmilk also provides the mildness needed by the gut during a time of illness - the adequate hydration; since it contains mostly water, and the nutrients to help aid faster recovery.

The suck cycle from let-down to fully fed: the hindmilk

Take this to be a depiction of a full feeding cycle from let-down to the end milk called 'hindmilk' which is full of fat. It will help you understand what's happening at each phase of the feed cycle. This will make for more effective breast-feeding.

The baby is hungry. You make sure you're in a comfortable sitting or lying position to feed. You attach him or her to your bare breast, achieving a good latch, then the baby begins to suck, and all the crying or restlessness calms down into a slow suck pattern. Suck-suck-suck, suck-suck-suck, suck-

suck- then, you feel that 'letting-down' sensation; a pressure which travels down quickly into your breasts, a pull, a fullness sensation, which eventually fills your breasts. You feel a fullness and a swelling within its contents; a heaviness, and the breasts are full, ready to feed your baby. **Then you notice your baby starts to gulp, and gulp. It changes from suck-suck-suck to suck-swallow, suck-swallow, suck-swallow, swallow, and a splutter, a withdrawing, and a cough (which occasionally depicts how much milk you have and the pressure of the let-down now influencing the fast pace of milk flow into your baby's mouth). Baby then quickly reattaches (assuming he has had an overflow into his mouth), still hungry, and regains a suck-swallow rhythm; all the while enjoying himself, showing some signs such as a jolly grabbing of his free leg with his free hand, a rubbing of your other breast, a rubbing of your face, a humming, a smile looking up at you, etc.** The sensation and the satisfaction for them is not solely from the breastmilk, but something deeply satisfying and stimulating about breastfeeding. It's a compulsory enjoyment for them at this age of their development.

The breasts were meant to be a centre of delight for them.

As breastfeeding draws to a close, the rhythm begins to change, with a few more sucks before a swallow, as the milk in the breasts continue to empty into your baby's mouth. If they are still hungry, evidenced by persistent sucks and no sign of wanting to come off, consider switching over to the other breast. They will find more there. Both breasts are filled at let-down, so baby has a top up container if still hungry after the first feed.

The breasts were meant to be a centre of delight for them.

As the breast empties, towards that terminal suck-suck swallow phase, where there are often a few more sucks before swallow, there comes a phase where they appear to be barely exerting their suckle and it feels more like a flutter of their tongue, followed by a swallow. This is the phase where the hindmilk is found. It is important to let them get the milk from this phase. Hind-milk differs in composition from the foremilk. It is high in fat, which fills out the baby's hollows. Here's what a GP notebook article on breastmilk says about the hindmilk:

> "Fat content in human breast milk is variable during the feed. Initially, the fat content of human milk is low and this rises to about 3% by the end of the feed."

As much as possible, try to ignore the temptation to rush through a breastfeeding session. Just enjoy it. One way to add enjoyment to your postpartum is to allow yourself enjoy and soak in the experience, just as your child does.

Don't rely solely on the suckles to tell when your child is getting the hindmilk. By allowing your child to feed and come off by themselves when full, you can be satisfied they're feeding fully. Occasionally, they sleep off and forget to come off. You can withdraw your nipple by gently inserting a washed and clean finger in between their gums, creating enough space between the gums to withdraw your nipple without grazing it against any hard surfaces. If they wake up and cling to your breasts and then try to come back on, let them if you can.

As the breast empties, towards that terminal suck-suck swallow phase, where there are often a few more sucks before swallow, there comes a phase where they appear to be barely exerting their suckle and it feels more like a flutter of their tongue, followed by a swallow. This is the phase where the hindmilk is found.

CHAPTER 5

CHALLENGES ALONG THE WAY THE SECOND TIME

Dealing with engorgement and blocked ducts

Due to the declarations I had made over myself - accidentally prophesying an excess into my experience, I believe it culminated in what I got.

Here's my experience:

On day 2/3, my breasts became much fuller. My milk had 'come in'. My baby lived on my breasts before then, i.e., through days 1 and part of day 2. She suckled regularly and I just let her, for these reasons:

1. I wanted to ensure I breastfed successfully with no obstructions this time.

2. I knew all I had in my breasts at this time was colostrum and that it was only produced in small quantities. I assumed this meant she would need to come on more frequently. I was prepared for this mentally. I was going to do whatever it took, including holding her up to my breasts all through day one; except when she was either asleep, or just coming off and fully settled.

So, I did this consistently until my milk came in the later part of day 2. What I experienced were:

✦ Fuller breasts; much fuller.

✦ Lumpiness. There were some lumps which felt more like solid or semi-solid areas in my breasts and could occasionally depress on applying pressure with a finger.

The quadrants of the breast could each experience engorgement. The breast comprises 4 quadrants, and this is useful for descriptive purposes. Also because some quadrants will be more likely to get engorged than others, depending on how your baby feeds and what areas he is more likely to drain from depending on the feeding methods used. The 'method' involves the feeding position, how you position your breasts for increased flow from certain areas, leaving out others, etc.

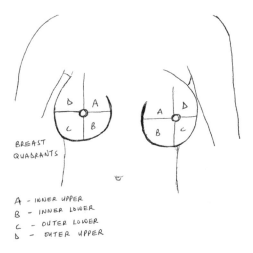

BREAST QUADRANTS

A - INNER UPPER
B - INNER LOWER
C - OUTER LOWER
D - OUTER UPPER

The inferior quadrants seemed to get engorged more frequently for me. This was because the top quadrants were more likely to be drained first in my feeding, leaving me to hand-press milk out of the inferior part of my breast, by feeding it out toward the direction of the nipple, and in this way guiding the milk out. Simply applying pressure on the engorged parts, or areas of blocked ducts, while letting the baby suckle at the nipple at the same time often resolved the blockade.

Other things I tried that provided some help for me were:

1. Applying a warm compress over the engorged/solidified areas. This seemed to soften lumps and aid milk outflow just before feeding.

2. **Changing from one position to try other positions which seemed to be more effective in draining other areas of the breast. It is very important to try feeding in different positions.**

By trying various positions, you will come to know of which positions work for you, both in providing of comfort for you and the baby, as well as draining the milk effectively. I discuss positions in the subsequent chapter. I was advised to take a warm shower, which worked to soften the breasts; softening the congealed milk within them (if I can use this term for milk still within the breasts). The problem was, in my case, I found the showers somehow caused increased milk let-down into my breasts, while also allowing the milk within it to flow. As such, it got the tap running both into as well as out of my breasts. Overall, this wasn't helpful for me. I seemed to have milk let-downs too often, in excess of how fast the baby could empty it. The build-up caused my breasts to swell in immense sizes. The look was astonishing; not only because of their storage capacity, which was reflected in how many times their normal size they had become, but also because of the shape change the lumps had caused.

The resulting pain was sometimes unbearable, and I would sometimes cry. This pain results from an inflammation of some of the tissue which has come into direct contact with the milk from the pressure inside the breasts, and also because of the skin stretching to the limits of capacity within a short time. This should not scare you. You may not suffer engorgement to this degree, but I did, so I can tell you the true extent of what it feels like, so that you would be armed with the knowledge of what to do in case you experienced it too. I had to call in the midwife, as I needed help beyond the home measures I knew. She linked me with other healthcare staff. So, I was sent into the hospital to see the healthcare staff, and after reviewing my history from pregnancy into puerperium, they asked me to latch baby onto my breasts so they could watch me feed. They wanted to assess my breastfeeding position, my technique, and baby's latch. They stated everything was as it should be, but they could observe I was in very obvious discomfort with the breastfeed. This caused them, after examining my lumpy engorged breasts, to retrieve their pump in an attempt to relieve me of some pressure. It was a hospital-grade milk extractor. I'd call it that. It did a good job of withdrawing the milk faster and much easier than my handheld medela pump.

They managed to drain off some milk from my breasts in the hospital. This provided little relief as unfortunately the breasts kept filling up as they drained them. She would come on to suckle on my engorged breast, and I would have a let-down to replace the amount she drained. The same with the hospital pump.

Things you can do to help relieve the pain and inflammation from engorgement are:

✦ *Take a mild NSAID (Non-Steroidal Anti-Inflammatory Drug):* The over-the-counter ones for everyday use are typically safe if you don't have any risk factors, such as taking another NSAID or pain killer for any other reason. Check with your healthcare provider in this case, if you don't have any history of peptic ulcer disease (an ulcer in your stomach) and are likely not to be advanced in age (which increases the risk from these kinds of medicines). That is, provided you're a fit and young adult, you should be able to have short-term (5-day course) or one-off use. It's always a good idea still, to check in with your doctor; you just may never know what concerns they may have or find relating to your case. So check. It's harmless and will be helpful for their record keeping. If you take NSAIDs, you want this to be on record, as it can help prevent complications with prescribing certain other treatments in the future. The information provided here is very general and of course, does not consider all that should ideally be considered in your particular case. Thus, it cannot be relied upon as direct medical advice.

✦ *Use Savoy Cabbage:* This I found to be very soothing. In fact, after it was told to me by the healthcare provider, I drove off straight from that breast-drain hospital appointment to a supermarket. I picked up some from the veggie section, rinsed it under running tap water once I got home, and stored it in the fridge for a couple of hours to cool down. When cooled, I peeled off outer wrap after outer wrap, inserting it over my breasts and into my bra as you normally would with a breast pad, and I let it cool my breasts and ease the inflammation. It provided a great deal of relief, providing cooling that was very soothing for my entire mind and breasts.

In my case, a short course of an NSAID and the use of the savoy cabbage helped me a great deal to provide relief. An anti-inflammatory agent was more helpful than a different class of analgesic because it dealt directly with inflammation, which was the issue. Ultimately, the permanent solution was my supply had to regularise to become just enough for the needs of my baby. So, I went back to the root I perceived to be the cause - my earlier declarations. I began to recall my statements earlier said. Because I thought, if by my declaration I have caused this overflow, surely the same power of my words would solve the problem. I then began speaking and commanding my supply to re-regulate to just meet my baby's demands; to be just sufficient and not overflow. I took back what I had thought to be a good breastfeeding prayer – an overflow, surplus. Not in this case. No, not with breastfeeding.

The exception to this would be if you plan on pumping and storing/freezing milk for later use, or maybe donating some milk.

Shivers

During the first weeks of my breastfeeding journey, while still dealing with engorgement and the likes, I noticed I would often shiver and feel unnecessarily cold.

This occurred with no other symptoms indicating something was wrong. A friend told me it happened to her also, and she suggested it might be because of the engorgement. I had no signs of infection anywhere. My boobs weren't red or hot, I didn't feel unwell or notice any fever. Just shivers and some chills. At that time, I was nursing round the clock, doing some housework, and helping to look after my older son. Hence, there was physical exertion, then the increased metabolic demands of breastfeeding, and I wasn't drinking enough water or eating as much as I should, unfortunately. I should have drunk a bit more water and eaten a bit more in retrospect. Fortunately, the shivers passed on their own without me needing any intervention. I never found out the definitive explanation for them.

I share these things because I'm trying to make you, the reader, a little more confident with your breastfeeding journey. Sometimes, simply knowing you're not the only one or the first to go through some difficulty with your journey arms you with the confidence to push through; especially when you see others who've gone through the same and have come through it successfully. That's what this book is about. It's not a 'Breastfeeding-is-a-smooth-journey-with-no-hurdles-book', but a 'One may face these challenges on their own journey, but can definitely come through all of them, and succeed' book. Hopefully, you won't have to face many of these, but if you do, know there's comfort and information available to you. This will make it less of an anxious road for you.

Dealing with excoriations & cracked nipples

Cracked nipples and nipple excoriations were the most challenging part of my journey. They are basically formed by the hard part of your baby's mouth grazing repeatedly against the skin around your nipples. It can be improved by a good latch and may also be improved by trying various positions and finding one that works. A good latch positions the nipple within the baby's mouth, in such a way that most of the force applied during suckling is by the soft palate and the tongue of your baby.

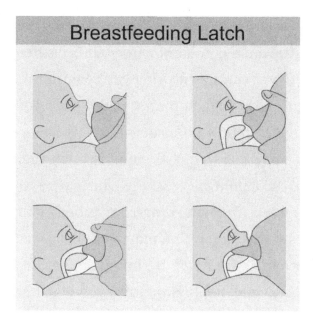

Breastfeeding Latch

You are more likely to get a good latch in certain positions than in others, dependent on the preference of you and your baby. The next chapter deals with breastfeeding positions. You can have a look through and try a couple as you go along, until you find one or a few that work for you.

This trauma induced nipple damage generally tends to last only the first few weeks and then naturally eases with healing as you find your rhythm. I had multiple tubes of nipple cream – I used a lanolin-based nipple cream and kept this at different points around the house for ease of access. I would layer this generously on top of my nipples after every feed, and place a breast pad over it, as I noticed the pain was much worse when the skin around the nipples was dry. The breast pad came between the broken skin and my clothing. The lubricant also made it easier to separate the nipples from the breast pad or bra when it was time to feed again. Broken skin otherwise tends to stick to things surrounding it, and can be tricky to peel off before a feed. My excoriations gradually healed and became less painful with subsequent feeds. When the baby's teeth starts to come in, also be careful with latching and unlatching. I did not have any issues with this, but sometimes this can cause grazing too. I would emphasise consistency with the nipple cream. Use it generously to cover all wounded areas as soon as feeding is finished. Don't worry about baby getting this into her mouth as they are made to be safe for this, so no need to go washing or cleaning the nipple before feeding. Don't worry, you've got this. You can definitely do it.

Dealing with dizziness from dehydration

I got up from bed one morning and felt so faint I had to lie back down. I lay down for a while, and then my baby wanted a feed. I knew I was hungry and would be better off getting some food in my body before attempting to breastfeed the baby; as I needed strength to feed her. This goes back to what I mentioned about responsive feeding being convenient for mum and baby. The idea is that you respond to their cues. Acknowledging, even when you're not able to attend to them immediately, is better than ignoring because you can't do anything about it at the moment.

On this day, I knew I needed to be fed first, as I hadn't eaten anything that morning, and was really thirsty. I had been feeling dizzy on sitting or standing up. Alarm bells had gone off in my mind and I knew I had to do something to rectify this situation immediately. I thought about the possibility of passing out from hypoglycaemia while breastfeeding or becoming too tired to even carry her for the feed, or too tired to complete the feed. I just didn't want to lose the capacity to care for her. This was a classic example of needing to care properly for yourself to care for another. We were also both alone at home at the time. I came down from the bed slowly and gradually, making use of everything my medical knowledge informed me of in this situation. I changed my position so slowly that I hoped I could somehow cope with the symptoms when standing. Even so, it was a challenge. I managed to get myself down to the kitchen and to some water, and I drank as much as I could, and ate some food quickly, then came back up to the baby, and picked her up to feed. My symptoms remained for a while, and then gradually faded away as I continued to hydrate. I knew enough never to let things get to that place again. I took a water bottle to bed with me every night, and began actively gauging my water intake, and monitoring the colour of my urine to gauge hydration.

Your relationship with God in this time: Gone with the wind?

This was a time when my normal schedule had gone with the wind and all things had become new. I slept in the morning, woke up at midday, slept at night, and would wake up at midnight or intervals during the early hours of the morning to feed baby, play with her, and watch her stare off and entertain herself during the early hours of the morning. I often felt very sleepy, and for me this was the second hardest thing, apart from having excoriated nipples. It didn't last too long, for in the third month, I discovered I could breastfeed lying down, which I will talk about in the coming pages.

While still in this phase, I would often miss my relationship with God. I expected to still be able to spend quiet time with Him, not acknowledging my current situation and the changes it would introduce. The feeling of being in charge of my schedule was missing. I missed having things in control and having structure, and one day, while I was missing all these things, and wondering if I was still useful to God in active service, God whispered to me and said something along these lines,

> *"Every new phase of life should be an opportunity to relate with me in a new way,*

to experience a new depth of relationship and dependence on me."

He continued,

"You can either let circumstances push you away, or you can use them to draw near in a new way."

God had not waited there (where I thought I left Him, in the structured quiet meeting place), He had followed me. He had come with me right into the 'mess' and was right there with me. He's not only a God of the smooth seasons. He knows how to put on boots and get down and dirty with us in the chaotic or simply 'different' phases of our lives. As such, we should relax and find out how He's relating with us in that season. Simply relax and re-establish relationship with Him in that season and quit trying to rush that season to return where you think you left God. Also, quit worrying so much that you don't enjoy what's right before you. You're going to go through it anyway, so why not find the beauty in it? Struggle to make yourself see the beauty in your present condition. No matter what you're going through, your experience out of it can be positive. Right here in this mess, you can have a great and beautiful relationship with God too. Quit looking back, and look onto His face, right here beside you; here in the now. Let Him go through it with you. When you can't pray; rest, sleep and trust Jesus to pray for you. He's always 'interceding' for us anyway. He's given His angels charge over all your affairs. They guard you day and night. You have just as much authority now as you did before. You are just as much loved right now, and just as much valued. Rest and let him take care of you.

Don't forget to enjoy the baby right before you. Rest comes from believing in Jesus to take care of you, and to cover for you on the battlefield, while you attend to your baby and be the best mum you can. So, taking the Holy Spirit's advice, I got Him involved, asked Him questions, spoke to Him while rocking my daughter during her crying periods - asking Him what to do, asking Him for suggestions or directions in areas where I had no idea. I trusted He knew the right way for every step. He had nature's key, so I asked Him. Because one thing was clear, I wanted all the right ways to get things done. For instance, I knew He'd know what was right for her skincare. He had the answer to the right hair care for her hair type. I brought Him in on all of those steps; often asking Him questions as I went. He gave me the idea of how to put together the hair care combination I now use, and her hair grew well. Soon after asking Him how to naturally produce the right hair care products to use on both our hairs, a friend from the locality came in one day, and I thought to ask her what she used on her daughter's hair, and she told me it was basically a mixture of natural products – specific plant based oils mixed with some shea butter, and I thought, this is down the same paths my thoughts have been leading me! I felt He had definitely led her there that day and had prompted me to ask her.

Much later, when my baby started showing signs of needing to feed on solids (just after her fourth month), my thoughts had started to go down the path of giving her natural foods and avoiding canned and manufactured foods. Coincidentally, I remembered a book I had owned with healthy baby food recipes in it, which I recommend by the way, (Annabel Karmel's Baby & Toddler Meal Planner). You can find it on Amazon. I had lent it to someone to help with her own baby when she had reached weaning age, and I now felt compelled to retrieve the book. I did, and started to have a look at it, and within it I saw the recipes were easy and I could easily make them using things I had in my fridge and kitchen. So I had a first try using an inspiration I had outside of the book for a meal made with beans boiled until soft. This is a local recipe, using black eyed beans boiled soft with some boiled plantains and then some steamed and seasoned mackerel fish. I pureed the above mixture, adding some mild fish stock, to create a soft consistency and offered this to her when she had just completed four months and was into her fifth month. I did not start solids earlier than this. This was her first meal. She ate the whole thing. I was awed. Before this, she had frequently tried to grab my food when I was eating; often batting at my cup whenever she saw me drinking. She showed an actual interest whenever she saw me eating and I took this to mean she was ready for solids, and I wasn't wrong. In addition, in her fourth month she had started to require milk more. It didn't seem to fill her for as long anymore and I was having to breastfeed more. I began giving her purees from the recipe book, making a variety of recipes with fruits and vegetables as stated in the book and also trying other recipes I found elsewhere. This turned out well. Most people choose instead to start giving formula at this stage, but that's not actually what their bodies are calling for. It just needs more satisfying nutrition. So far, she has generally not been a picky eater and will try almost everything we eat. I believe breastfeeding influences the ease with which a child will get on to its parents' usual foods. I also believe delaying getting onto solid foods does nothing good for the baby.

I have shared my story in this way to give you a well-rounded picture of everything that played a part. I have shared about God and my relationship with Him because He played an undeniable part. To leave Him out would give an incomplete story and would deny Him His necessary credit.

Weaning

This is not meant to teach you how to wean or to explore all the different methods of weaning there are, as I simply write from my perspective, and advocate what I've seen work well. What I would like to emphasise here is giving natural foods when you start to wean. I advocate eating a nutritious diet yourself, as this will tell on what she gets in breast milk. The NHS recommends exclusive breastfeeding for six months. I personally chose to start earlier as from the signs that I saw, I felt that she was ready for feeds. And she really proved that she was by how she gobbled the first meal and how easily her gut handled it and she thrived on it.

When I started weaning my child, it was a plant-based diet at first. I made sure to make it myself, using the cookbook I mentioned earlier from Annabel Karmel and some online recipes. I would puree different mixtures of fruits and/or vegetables. The book also provides step-by-step information you can find useful on how to go about weaning and behavioural changes to expect at the different ages.

+ I often gave her things I didn't like or wasn't accustomed to eating myself, such as certain vegetables; so that I wouldn't limit her based on my own tastes.

+ I learnt to introduce her to different tastes, including sour foods, so that she would become comfortable eating non-sweet things.

What eating home-made foods did was allow us to avoid the chemical preservatives in store-bought foods. *I believe this period is just as important as deciding to breastfeed.*

I advocate breastfeeding, and then feeding homemade foods for the period of weaning. It's fine if you have the occasional store-bought preparation. Certain periods of convenience may require this. Home-made preparations can be made in large batches and stored in small storage containers. I will advise you use a recipe book for continued supply of ideas. This will save you money from having to buy the pre-made meals, as well as encourage the optimal growth and healthiness of your child. I'll will show why this is important later. As part of their milestones, you will notice when they start to reach for the spoon to feed themselves. Encourage it. This is their auto-biology clock saying it's time to start self-feeding, but often some parents either don't pick up on it or don't yet want the mess that comes with it so they don't encourage it. When you notice them starting to do certain things or show interest in new actions, it's good to encourage them to practise that action until they perfect it. Examples are when they reach for cutlery to self-feed, or when they reach for your food as you eat i.e., before you've started weaning, or swat your cup towards themselves when they see you drink, when they attempt to stand, or walk, attempt to talk or imitate your movements. Give it meaning, explore it further with them.

When they show interest, capitalise on it to establish the skill at that time. That's nature's way of highlighting they're due and ready to start that new thing, and your role would be to teach and support them in establishing that skill.

Overcome the temptation to force feed.

This was something I had to learn myself. "Don't force-feed her" were the words whispered in my ears as my frustration piled up while trying to feed her one day. I recognised the voice that spoke to me. His voice carried both the message and its meaning. I intuitively understood the reason I should not force food on her, and no one captures it better than these few paragraphs of the book 'My Child Won't Eat' by Carlos Gonzalez. In the foreword for his book, Professor Amy Brown explains,

> "It is normal for babies and young children to go through stages where they refuse to eat certain foods or seemingly exist on thin air from barely eating a thing. Refusing to try new foods is likely protective – after all we would not want our newly mobile babies to crawl off to the nearest poisonous berry bus and eat them all. Few babies and children will willingly starve themselves. More likely they are simply more masterful at listening to their internal cues of what their body needs – something many adults will recognise they have sadly lost."

She says,

"The second thing to remember is that your baby's early experiences around food are important. Not in terms of what they do or do not eat, but their social and emotional experiences around eating. We all have our own personal memories and connotations of different foods. Where did they come from? From our early experiences of how they were shared with us. Were we encouraged to try them or were we forced to eat them before we could leave the table? Were mealtimes strict or were they a chance to share love and connection with others as we enjoyed our food? Were all foods presented equally as part of a balanced, varied diet or were we told certain foods were a reward for enduring others?"

These paragraphs sum up the reason behind avoiding force-feeding in early childhood, as those memories go a long way to shape our eating habits even into adulthood. The book 'My Child won't eat' by Carlos Gonzalez is one I highly recommend amongst other books for child upbringing recommended in the last chapter.

During their six to twelve months, infections and other illnesses may start to appear. This is because the maternal immunity transferred at birth has waned, and they now have to fight by themselves, generating their own immunity. Even though the mother still supports by sending in some fighter cells through her breastmilk (if the child is continuing to breastfeed), the child is mostly responsible for developing its own immunity; as such they must be prepared and equipped for this. The world outside is full of all kinds of germs and disease causing bugs which are constantly adapting and trying to trick us (via mutations), and you will do very well to ensure they are as equipped for this stage as they can be. An important contributor at this time will be their diet – from breastfeeding exclusively, to weaning them at the right time; adding in a wide variety of fruits and vegetables to their diet - exposing them to various tastes, and also to animal foods, if your diet includes this.

Imagine this: Would you be willing to feed on store-bought ready-made foods and highly processed foods, stored with preservatives, or made from non-natural ingredients, as your main meals every day? How long do you think you could do this for? How would it then affect your tastes for natural foods? If you wouldn't, should we be feeding them in this way? I appreciate it's more convenient and almost a lifesaver for some families, but I wonder if we are actually doing the right thing for these little ones? I think **occasional** ready-made store-bought meals are fine so long as their diet is mostly healthy and made both cautiously and deliberately. This guarantees content, and absence of the harsh chemical ingredients which are likely harmful for their developing organs.

Just to add, I think screen time (if excessive) can reduce a child's opportunity for cognitive development, and the development of the child's imagination. Personally, I have not found the need to engage my daughter using screen time so far. In her free time, she plays about the house; exploring different items around the house, and playing with what she can find. I make it a habit to examine and ensure that whatever she chooses to play with is safe for her.

Only do the best you can. Some of this may take more from you, but it is infinitely worth the effort it takes, looking back. The gratitude one feels having known they put in their best is priceless. Thus, I'd recommend you start now to equip yourself with what you need to know; just as you're already doing and then move forward and give it the best you can. You would be glad you did.

Next, I delve into the subject of feeding positions, co-sleeping with your child and the dangers of it, as well as the other side to it I saw which marked the end of a certain gloom during my journey, and was a major turning point from the tiring insomnia during the first weeks.

CHAPTER 6

BREASTFEEDING POSITIONS FOR LESS STRESS: IS CO-SLEEPING SAFE?

A breastfeeding position adopted should be comfortable, secure, and enable you to get and hold the baby in a good latch for an effective feed. Below are the positions that worked the best for me, as well as others you can also try. The key is to try different positions until you find what works best. You can change positions even within a feed, especially if the current position hurts or is uncomfortable.

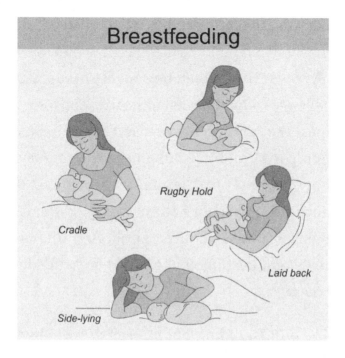

For me, the most suitable to start with was 'Rugby hold'. Positions may have different names in different resources, but they basically describe the same positions.

This was also something I didn't have in my first pregnancy - the guts or guidance to try out different positions; to try to find something that worked for me. I tried a few, and those without confidence, mostly because I didn't know breast-feeding could pose that much resistance.

> *This was also something I didn't have in my first pregnancy - the guts or guidance to try out different positions; to try to find something that worked for me.*

My mindset wasn't prepared to push past resistance, or persevere. So when I met challenges, it was easy to give up as I didn't realise there could be a reality of success beyond those challenges. I hadn't seen or heard of anyone who had pushed past the same challenges and come out successful. I was unprepared, and this influenced the course and outcome of my journey. I had assumed it would just flow naturally, since it was such a natural thing. I did not assume any challenges would be faced at all. And this mum said the same when questioned about her breastfeeding experience. She says:

> *"The mindset I had about breastfeeding was that it was going to be smooth. I read things online and saw people breastfeeding, like there was nothing to it."*
> *- Mum I.D.*

This is part of what informed this book. To show a mum what challenges they may face, and how to overcome them, or mostly that they CAN overcome them. I also aim to show in the latter parts of the book, why this is all so worth it in retrospect. I've been glad I held on in my case, because the results at the end are nothing short of amazing. And having a healthy, happy, well-developed child is one of the greatest blessings anyone could ask for. Knowing that you have done your part to give them the best start, and indeed the head start to their journey in life, brings fulfilment and I'd love for you to also feel that.

In my baby's month three, I moved on from mostly using the rugby hold with a pillow placed under her to prop her up, to feeding her in a lying down position with her lying beside me. (I found using a normal soft pillow more comfortable than a marketed breastfeeding pillow, because of the flexibility of the soft pillow).

This was when I started to sleep 'through' the night, only waking up to latch her on when she wanted to feed. Even so, this personally didn't feel like much of a disruption to my sleep as I didn't have to change from the lying position or get up from bed. She would feed and fall back asleep, and I would sleep too. I know about the worries with co-sleeping, but this is what I believe, and hear me out. In regional areas of the world, where 'traditional' ways of doing things have been preserved; i.e., in the sense of continuing things to a large extent with how they started, co-sleeping is still very much a major practice. We also see this in the fact that they recognize and naturally submit to a baby's requirement and displayed need to be close to its parent and primary caregiver during night sleep. A baby may want to feed at intervals through the night, and apart from their nutritional requirement, the comfort, shelter, and protection provided by having a human body in proximity during sleep is provided by its mother or caregiver (e.g., for an adopted child). This is the same feeling as a newlywed wife wanting to be near her husband during sleep. This is the same desire or need people have to snuggle up beside each other, especially in cold weather. We are all created with an innate need to have human warmth and comfort, especially during sleep. What this provides is a sense of security, shelter, and comfort; the same for the little one.

Most mothers will also naturally feel most comfortable when their babies are in proximity. The attempt at making beside-me cribs, which naturally flow into the adult bed recognise this need, but still it falls slightly short I must admit. I understand the concerns around this, and I deeply empathise with all the situations where harm has come from this. We must, however, also not forget to emphasize and continue to state the reason nature made it to be this way, that the mother provides warmth and the comfort from her proximity during night sleep.

Instead of prohibiting everyone, thereby cutting short the experience for those who would have safely given the bonding experience this affords to their little ones, and have in turn benefitted from the peace of mind and improved sleep, less stress, less needing to wake up and leave the bed at night that this affords, I propose a slightly different approach. **The approach I would advise is simply to**

state the truth: that co-sleeping is natural and the way it is originally supposed to be, and then I would heavily highlight the dangers posed by this modern world and our current way of life, and highlight all the situations people find themselves in that would pose an even greater danger to co-sleeping with your baby. The baby's safety should be paramount.

If you have smoked, drunk alcohol or any other liquid with the potential to influence your consciousness and ability to reason optimally, if you are under the influence of medication, you're injured or of reduced mobility for other reason, if you're a heavy sleeper or known to roll over and throw limbs about during sleep, if you have a parasomnia (a sleeping disorder e.g. sleepwalking), or anything at all that reduces your ability to be in your normal functioning subconscious mind during sleep, then co-sleeping isn't safe and I wouldn't advise it; because our priority should be to keep your baby safe. A baby is a vulnerable young human who has been entrusted to your care for safekeeping and rearing, so if you're compromised, look after their wellbeing by what I call the next best option, which is now mainstream in our day, i.e., placing them in their own cot, beside your bed in the same room. Having them in the same room still provides some proximity. Does this make sense? That is how I would state the matter, and I hope it provides some light and balance.

Extra pressures of this world we live in have also made it difficult, even often unrealistic, for mothers to follow the natural order. It often puts women under the pressure and demand to go back to work too early, in order to aid with catering for their families; whether work outside of the house or even normal housework which can be very hectic without help. All of this, the world exerting the pressure of its demands on us, has left us with no option but often to adapt the way we raise and nurture our babies to meet the demands of the world. So, we will get them off feeding at night, we get them out of our rooms early, try to teach their little developing minds to self soothe through the night and not need mummy, etc. Of course, mummy has to work and cope with other pressures in this world. Where everyone is physiologically normal and functioning optimally, nature designed for babies to sleep close to their mothers. That is to be mentioned, to raise the awareness of people who may not know this (and can afford to safely co-sleep) because of society prioritising all newer sleep structures for the new-born.

The earliest recorded history of a child coming to harm by sleeping close to its mother was in the case of a prostitute in the days of Solomon, the King, (who became king in the year 970 BC) recorded in the Bible (1 Kings 3: 16-28). She had rolled over, laid on and pressed her child in her sleep, until the child died; and then she exchanged the dead child for the child of another woman lying beside her in the same room during the night. It wouldn't be unreasonable to infer that this woman likely also had other situations compromising her health and making it unsafe for her care for the child. This story also shows that co-sleeping happened as far back as 3000 years ago, from the early ages. It's a very old concept, and the original way things happened back then. However, the limited safety in the current world cannot be denied too.

CHAPTER 7
BETTER OUTCOMES THE SECOND TIME AROUND

What I enjoyed the most the second time around was the bonding experience. Breastfeeding afforded the unique opportunity to bond with my child in a way nothing else could. It was delightful. One mum describes her own experience like this,

"If there was one thing I enjoyed the most about breastfeeding, it was the bonding experience. My child holding me very closely with her tiny hands, looking into my eyes, and smiling up at me when she was filled and dozing off with the milk dribbling from the corner of her mouth... And even now, we still have a very good bond"
- I.D.

Mummy D.A also mentions,

"The first few days I fed my son, he stationed his eyes on my face everytime like some art project. I have some pictures from that period that remain precious to date.'

She was reunited with her son after an initial brief period spent in the NICU. A third mum had this to say about the bonding with her children,

"If I had to do it again, if I had to breastfeed another child, I would, because it's really worth it. It's worth all the sleepless nights and all the stress."
- Mum T.K.

The process is enjoyable for both mother and child. A baby learns trust at its mother's breast. Comfort and security follow. A combination of breastfeeding and responsive care provision shapes its mind and perspective of the world for trust and security. I strongly believe this. We also see the ability of the immune system to mount up a more robust defensive in response to attack or invasion by microorganisms. Breast milk carries with it a taste of what you have eaten. This is the first exposure a child gets to its mother's diet, and so it should be easier technically speaking, to adapt the child onto your foods. Introducing solid foods on time also helped. Language and other forms of communication (nonverbal) developed faster and in correct context. Motor milestones came on solidly. Problem solving was good.

It was a beautiful journey, and I am especially thankful to God for giving me the strength and ability to push through all the hurdles and to get to experience the loving feedback that comes with breastfeeding. It is a blessing indeed. I hope you get to have the same, or an even better and smoother story.

CHAPTER 8

REDEMPTION; IF YOU HAVEN'T DONE IT PROPERLY WITH A PAST CHILD.

(My Redemption Story)

Results of early nurture

Are there any areas of their general development you have a problem with? Do you suspect that the early nurture as described so far in this book could have contributed to this? All is not lost, however, and long-lasting changes can begin to be made at any age in life. So, redemption is achievable and possible.

What I started to do once my eyes were opened to better ways of doing things:

1. Renew the diet: Changing the paths. This means renewing your diet too, and then your child's, to inculcating healthier foods.

Eat nature's foods. We all want to be healthy in the latter parts of our life. Oh well, the journey to that starts now. It's also really amazing how quickly things start to turn around when we start to make necessary changes.

Here are some tips I found useful:

1. Incorporating more vegetables and fruits into my diet.

2. Not overcooking vegetables - first learning how each one should be cooked to preserve as many nutrients within, and then proceeding to apply this learning to my food preparation methods.

3. Growing herbs at home.

4. Trying to limit to the barest minimum, or as much as is possible, all exposure to environmental toxins, e.g., cutting down on use of plastic for food storage, or merely being aware of the danger of this with plastic leaching

into the food when non-food-safe plastic is used. The ones labelled food safe may be safer for use.

- Also, just being aware of the safety issues surrounding microwaving food and trying as much as possible to reduce the heat/temperature used to cook foods; being aware that this can change or alter the composition of certain foods. My aim is to produce a mindset shift, because then all other changes can stem from that. Simply getting the awareness of these things is enough to start.

- Also, being aware of the preservative load of our foods, especially commercially bought pre-made meals.

5. Knowing the effects a lack of exercise or a sedentary lifestyle can have on us.

6. The degree to which a lack of a proper sleep routine or not getting enough sleep constantly can change or hamper the development of the healing systems and immune system in our bodies. This can also negatively influence memory, concentration, and mood.

7. Lastly, awareness of how the stress response mechanisms we have can affect things. Developing better stress coping mechanisms makes a great deal of

difference for overall health, and we should teach this to our children too. I get mine from Philippians 4:6-7 where it says "Be anxious for nothing, but in everything by prayer and supplication, with thanksgiving, let your requests be made known to God; and the peace of God which surpasses all understanding, will guard your hearts and minds through Christ Jesus."

These are some things I learned by reading, learning from others, and researching myself once my attention was drawn to the need for healthier lifestyles for me and my entire family.

So, here are some questions I asked myself:

✦ How much sleep are my kids getting? And are they getting enough? How much sleep should each one be getting at their stage of development? This information is available to be researched and implemented right away.

✦ How much exercise as physical activity do they need to get every day?

✦ How is my stress management? What does my stress response look like? Am I 'flail-flabbergasted-dishevelled' or calm-and-rational in my response to stress? There is a process to get here. It's a journey to this place.

+ Do I have a positive outlook to life/perspective/way of processing things? And subsequently, am I teaching this to my children too?

+ Do the children seem to give up easily on new tasks? Or get too emotional when not able to complete a task? E.g., get frustrated and cry or yell.

+ Do they seem to need excessive or constant affirmation to keep them assured of their abilities when they face challenges?

I will list some easy resources I have found very great use in. They help with beginning to make some simple changes. Anyone could easily adopt most of the changes, so don't worry. At the end of the day, what we want are healthy kids who we know we've done our best for. Change can really start at any age. Yes, any age, and can still have an effect and make a difference, although the later you start the more effort it might require; but it is still accomplishable. So, this is not about blaming, but recognising what may not be going well and seeing how you can change it. Reading books and educating myself on how the mind and brain of a child functions and develops, and what they need to aid their development, has made a tremendous impact on my parenting. With greater understanding comes better nurture. I believe other parts of the nurture my first time around could have affected the different outcomes, rather than just a choice of whether to breastfeed or persevere with breastfeeding alone.

These are some books I have found helpful so far:

+ The Whole Brain Child by Dr Daniel J. Siegel and Dr Tina Payne Bryson.
+ Happy Children (A step-by-step parenting guide) by Pia W. Davies.
+ My Child Won't Eat by Carlos Gonzalez
+ I also learned about the mind-gut connection from the book titled 'The Mind-Gut Connection' by Emeran Mayer, MD. It showed how the diet we expose ourselves and kids to, can affect our immune function, mood, decision making, and long-term health. This applies tangibly to our children.

These are just written resources. Of course, there have been many other forms of learning as resources become more easily seen once you develop an interest in them.

Fixing relationships:

One benefit of breastfeeding is it kick-starts the bonding between mother and child early. If for any reason you feel like the healthy bond between your child and you is lacking, if they seem detached or excessively un-reliant, here are some tips I found useful:

1. Spending quality time together. i.e., time doing something you both enjoy. It is important that you enjoy it, as well as your child, and that you really allow yourself to have fun while doing it. This will keep you from getting absent minded or impatient while at it.

2. Physical contact: Hugs and kisses.

3. Conversations: Conversations where you see the child's reasoning and learn how their mind works, where you listen, really listen and rub minds, teach them, transfer knowledge.

When a child feels heard, it can really bring about bonding. Also, when you're able to get down to their level and speak in a way they're likely to understand, this fosters bonding and transference of knowledge, which is how they really start to look like you in thinking. This transference of reasoning, from you to your child, is one form of mentorship between a mother or father and a child.

Thankfully, we can correct things and bring about some positive change at whatever point we pick up the mantle or responsibility to begin to do so. It will just require more intentional work and the restructuring of your life to make sure you've got the resources to nurture your children in the way they should go. But if you leave with one thing, know it is doable and you can be a successful parent!

Good luck.

CHAPTER 9
PASSING THE KNOWLEDGE ON

Hello mum, I wanted to share this idea with you to help other mums who like I was, are starting off their own journeys, or are repeating the journey but aren't fresh. Or just anyone whom you know would be better off having this and some other knowledge to help them on their journey. Try this:

1. Give them a book on breastfeeding (this, if you've found it useful), as one of their baby shower or newborn baby gifts. Probably better they get it before delivery.

2. For a more personalised additional gift with some love, get our pregnancy journal. This is a blank book with sheets where you can write personalised notes and

all the tips you remember from your own experience. Our pregnancy specific journal created just for this purpose is titled **'All I've Learned from Pregnancy and Postpartum'** and can be found for purchase on Amazon.

I want to create a culture where ladies feel comfortable sharing knowledge and passing it down. There would be so much less anxiety, ignorance and feeling of loneliness in the postpartum period if this became a common thing. These will make thoughtful, and really impactful gifts for whoever gets them. Happy reading to the mum who receives these!

All I've Learned from Pregnancy and Postpartum

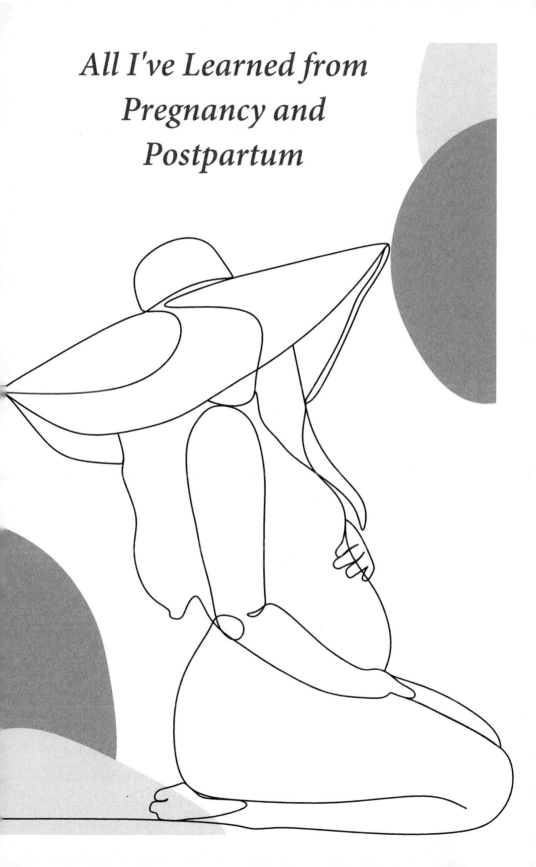

DISCLAIMER

I have not written this book totally as a medical doctor giving medical advice, but as a girl who had difficulty starting breastfeeding, failing at it the first time, and succeeding at my second opportunity through perseverance, doggedness, and God's help.

Because this is not a medical textbook, rather information from experience put together and backed up by research, I have not visited every condition, and unfortunately this did not cover every hiccup a woman might face on her breastfeeding journey; because I wanted to write from personal experience and compassion in my heart. My personal experience informed these things, backed up by research.

I encourage you to read other books written on the subject just as I did and found helpful. Everyone writes from a different perspective, and you arm yourself with a widespread breath of experience by reading different books. However, if you aren't able to, one is better than none. So well done.

Even if this were a medical book on the subject, I would still highly recommend that you look through other books, to compare knowledge, and help fortify the knowledge you've gained. This is because the breastfeeding stage is such a fundamental and quick stage of life, compared to the rest of one's life. And yet it is still so profound and key to the total health of your baby, that you want to ensure you're well prepared and fortified with the knowledge and help you need to give it the best shot you can.

Printed in Great Britain
by Amazon

18507099R00079